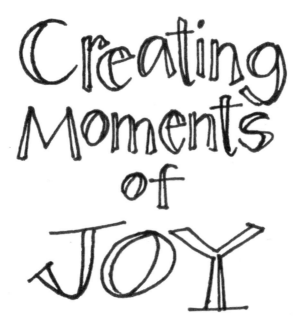

Creating Moments of JOY

Along the Alzheimer's Journey

Jolene Brackey

Fifth Edition

Purdue University Press, West Lafayette, Indiana

KH

I would like to gratefully acknowledge all of the writers I have quoted for their wisdom and inspirational words. If there is an error concerning permission to reprint, I apologize and a correction will be made in subsequent editions.

Cataloging-in-Publication Data is on file with the Library of Congress.

Paper ISBN: 9781557537607
ePDF ISBN: 9781612494821
ePUB ISBN: 9781612494838

This book is sold with the understanding that neither the author nor the publisher is engaged in tendering legal, accounting, medical, or other professional advice. If such advice or other assistance is required, the personal services of a competent professional should be sought.

9/15/17

Beloved is the Man
no one sees

Contents

Challenging Moments

Acknowledgments

People with Alzheimer's—*Thank you for teaching me*

Nutty Caregivers—*You are my inspiration*

Linda and Natalie—*Friends and "experts" on Alzheimer's*

Sisters of Providence—*Angel wings surrounding me*

Friends at Purdue—(^_^)

Friends at home—*Dance when the music plays*

Family—*Love my roots*

Freddy—*Filler of many cups*

Troy—*Steady cool water for this flower*

Sidnee—*Gypsy artist…lava*

Taylor—*Butterfly fly high*

Keegan—*Who knows me better than you?*

Stacie—*Queens for a life*

Mom and Dad—*For giving me wings to fly*

A mountain of gratitude to ALL who polished this gem:
Sister Ellen, Sister Ruth, Sister Mary Rita, Kelley, and, of course, Dustin.

Peter, this was dug up again only because you asked and
graciously offered your monkey wisdom throughout.

A sweet long embrace to Stacie—my niece, friend, and
steady rock. My goodness we make a magical team.

Bless our labor of love.

How to Use This Book

I have a vision. A vision to look beyond the challenges of Alzheimer's and focus on creating moments of joy. With short-term memory loss life is made up of moments. There are not perfectly wonderful days; there are perfectly wonderful moments—moments that put a smile on their face and a twinkle in their eye. Five minutes later, the person will have forgotten what was said and done; the feeling, however, lingers on. This new edition of *Creating Moments of Joy* is sprinkled with hope, fueled with wisdom, and lightened with humor. Our greatest teacher is the person with Alzheimer's, and who we explore is…Ourselves.

 Defining Moments—Signs that tell you it's time.

 Family Moments—This section will help you understand the strain the caregiver feels and how we, together, can support those giving care.

 Challenging Moments—This is a difficult journey, one you did not ask for. May this section teach you little tricks to lighten the load.

 Transitioning Moments—You will encounter many transitions as the person moves through this disease. Learn how to sustain and trigger memories along the way.

 Enhanced Moments—In each moment there is an opportunity to create a better moment. Discover how.

 Final Moments—May we all grow spiritually and cherish the teachings along the way.

Keep it simple. Open the book to one chapter that speaks to you. You will make mistakes. Mistakes are treasures too because they teach you what not to do. With short-term memory loss you get many "do-overs," and each moment is a new moment. As a family, scribble notes everywhere about anything at all; one person can write with a blue pen, another with red, and another with black. When the time comes, pass on this book filled with your struggles and solutions so wants and wishes are not lost, but bound together.

Every person with Alzheimer's is completely different. Therefore, I am not your teacher; your experience with this person, in each moment, is your teacher.

It's also my true desire to create moments of joy for you, the person who holds and reads this book. I have carefully selected stories, quotes, and dashes of humor—may you remember, cry, laugh, love, and find a bit of hope.

Knowledge is the foundation of Wisdom, but Wisdom means nothing unless you apply it. —THE BUNNY

Prelude

Bob was an avid fly fisherman and loved fishing the streams of Oregon. I met him when he moved into our community after being diagnosed with Alzheimer's. Bob had a wonderful relationship with his wife, and I asked her to bring me one of his fishing poles. We were all outside enjoying the sun when his wife opened the door with a fishing pole in her hand. I gave the pole to Bob and asked if he would show us how to cast. He tossed the line out with such ease—and then handed me the fishing pole. Needless to say, I didn't do very well, but he enjoyed watching me try. Then I asked him, "How do you tie the lures on?" He grabbed into the air for a fishing line, which wasn't really there, and he moved his hands and fingers as if he were tying the knot. He looked over at me with the imaginary knot in his hand and a smile on his face. I said, "You're amazing." And he just laughed.

This is what I mean by "creating a moment of joy." Bob relived a beloved pastime: fly-fishing. If his wife had not brought his fishing pole, this moment would not have occurred. We would have missed our opportunity to create a moment of joy. Instead, we captured it. We created a moment of joy for the people who lived in our community, for me, for Bob's wife, and, most importantly, for Bob.

Defining Moments

The moon reveals a whole new light. —JOLENE

Signs

We were playing cards and mom always kept score. Mom handed the score pad to me. She couldn't keep score anymore.

My husband and I taught ballroom dance. Before dance class began, he asked me, "What are we doing here?"

My dad and brothers went hunting. My dad dropped off my brothers and said he'd pick them up down the road, but he went home and forgot all about them.

My husband was always good with money and did our finances. One day I discovered we were actually in the red. He had not been subtracting the money correctly in the checkbook.

My mother was an awesome baker but she could no longer follow a recipe.

He looked at our grandson and said, "You have got to take care of the pigs." We didn't have pigs anymore and he thought he was talking to our son.

We took Mom out to eat and she couldn't zip her coat. Plus, she couldn't do the kids' puzzles on the back of the menu as she always had.

My cousin went elk hunting with my husband like they always did each year. My husband noticed odd things like my cousin taking all of the food out of the cooler, or leaving the lantern on all the time. Then my cousin just wandered off into the woods. Fortunately he took the walkie-talkie with him so my husband was able to call him on it and ask him where he went, to which my cousin replied, "I don't know." My husband did find him and they were able to safely make it home. We talked with my cousin's wife about what happened and she just said, "Oh, I thought he would have said something to you about it since you're so close with him."

I moved in with my grandma after my grandpa passed away. There were reminder notes everywhere and I didn't think anything of it until we went to Las Vegas together. She lost her bus pass three times. We went out to eat and the total was $6.75. After looking through her money awhile, she handed the cashier $105.24. I told my dad but he didn't want to hear about it and made excuses for her. It only became worse. She missed paying bills, paid them twice, or wrote checks for the wrong amount. I finally convinced my dad to take her to the doctor. At that point he discovered she was spending large amounts of money on random things. There were many signs over five years, but my family was in denial. I made Grandma's appointment, and even after she was diagnosed my family made excuses about why she failed the test. They continued to let her live at home alone and drive for another six months. I wish I would've been more persistent, but I'm only the granddaughter.

Early detection is key. Consider doing a memory screening every year so you can plan ahead instead of waiting for a catastrophic moment.

God gives his hardest battles to his strongest soldiers. —HELEN KELLER

Newfound Sign

Get a Diagnosis

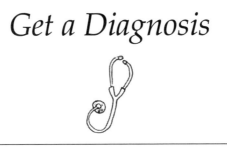

Written by an individual affected by Alzheimer's.

A definitive diagnosis of Alzheimer's is not yet possible until an autopsy is performed. But neural testing can be done that indicates the likelihood of whether Alzheimer's, or a related dementia, is the root cause of the problem. There are other diseases, like Parkinson's for instance, that can have symptoms similar to those of Alzheimer's, so don't assume anything. Consult with a doctor.

It's surprising how many people *know* something is wrong and yet do nothing about it. Then there are those who remain in willful (or fearful) denial, making excuses for, or hiding, the symptoms of a real problem. In this first instance, perhaps they think that by ignoring the issue it will just go away. In the second, it is as if denying the existence of the problem will somehow make it not real. *No.* A broken bone is a broken bone, whether you ignore it, try to will it unbroken, wish it unbroken, or make believe it is not broken. Seeing a doctor about a problem won't make it any more or less real—it is what it is—but it *will* enable you to make informed choices about what you need to do next.

How many times have you witnessed a mole-sized problem turn into a mountain-sized one due to inaction? For this very reason, address issues as soon as you become aware of them.

Often people assume the worst and fear having their assumptions verified. Well if they already assume the worst, it wouldn't be a shock if it actually *is* the worst. But what if it isn't as they fear? Then they'd have reason to be relieved. That can happen only *if* they actually go to the doctor and get checked out. If we find the courage to face them, often we'll discover the monsters of our imagination to be far bigger than the monsters of our reality.

Two good reasons to get a diagnosis:

1. To get a handle on it early on if it is something curable. If it is something incurable (like Alzheimer's), then there is time to prepare, make decisions as to future treatment (if any), and get affairs in order.

2. To give family and friends time to prepare themselves for this journey.

Keep in mind that the first doctor the person sees will most likely not be a specialist. Ask for a referral to a specialist to get a second opinion.

Late in life, my mom married a doctor and lived a fairytale life, or so it seemed. There was nothing she couldn't do. She skied until she was seventy and walked across the Golden Gate Bridge at seventy-five.

When my Mom turned eighty she decided to quit driving. We were stunned. We could see something was going on but thought surely our mother's husband, the doctor, had her health under control.

This is where the denial came in. He had hidden her illness from us for many years—in my opinion to preserve his own dignity—preventing us from helping her in any way. She was down to ninety-three pounds when we finally intervened without his blessing. To say the least he was verbally abusive to all of us, but it became no choice. It was explained to us by a professional that he was treating "his last patient." Sadly, it was not until her final years that were we able to give her the care she deserved. —ANNE

Recently my father-in-law, who has Alzheimer's, went missing for five days and was found four hours away severely dehydrated. Even after being told by the doctor he could no longer drive, my husband and mother-in-law refused to take his keys away. My mother-in-law talks about him like he's not there, and my husband won't talk to him because he doesn't want to upset him. He was in the hospital for a week and now they want to bring him back home, even though she is unable to care for him. They are in denial about how bad it is. —A DAUGHTER-IN-LAW

Denial is the root cause of inaction, and inaction can be dangerous.

If you worry about what might be, and wonder what might have been, you will ignore what is. —UNKNOWN

Newfound Diagnosis

Early Stages

R ealize that the early stages are the most difficult for the person with Alzheimer's, and quite frankly for the spouse, who is not yet the caregiver. Often in the early stages, the spouse thinks the person is doing these forgetful things on purpose, which causes resentment and frustration for even the strongest of couples. Once the spouse realizes it's the disease, the difficult journey of acceptance and change begins.

In the early stages, the person *knows* something isn't right. When they *feel* this, it may come through as sheer anger, panic, or sadness, but the honest undercurrent is the feeling of fear. They are afraid.

A common question is, "Do I tell the person they have Alzheimer's?"

June is a caregiver for her husband and feels that this approach provided her husband with some comfort: He asked, "What's wrong with me?" I told him, "You have dementia." "Is there a cure?," he asked. "They are working on it."

Ron has never asked what is wrong with him. He acts like nothing is wrong, only that he is getting old and forgetful. I think he knows something is wrong, but he has always been such a strong person and admitting that something is wrong would show weakness. —A WIFE

No two people are alike, each person goes through this journey in his or her own way. If they ask, then, yes, tell them *one* time the truth of what is happening. But if they don't bring it up, please *do not* remind the person. When you see the fear, reassure them: "This isn't your fault; you didn't create this. I'm not going anywhere and we will do this together." Allow them to *feel* what they are feeling. Let them vent. Rest assured this too shall pass, because in the middle stages the person doesn't think anything is wrong with them. It gets easier for them because they don't remember that they don't remember.

You—the spouse, the partner, the lover, the daughter, the son, the friend, the one who has chosen to walk with this person—allow yourself to feel *all* you are feeling. The plans you have made, the dreams you hoped to fulfill, and the supposed "golden years" are now blurry and unknown. Don't try to figure it out. Instead, feel what you are feeling in each present moment and gently move forward.

Allow *all* involved to feel what they are feeling. Just know that after we scream, after we cry, and after we shake it all out, we feel better. When the person with Alzheimer's screams, cries, or becomes quiet, it isn't personal. It isn't against you. Just give them space to be. There can be a tremendous amount of healing when we allow ourselves and others to feel what we are feeling. People simply need a safe place to land. A safe place to feel the feeling.

The amazing thing about life is that there are so many versions of yourself you get to experience. —STACIE

Newfound Expression

Understanding
the Person

Think of something from your childhood that makes you feel good just thinking about it: a wooden swing hanging from a tree, Grandma baking bread in the kitchen, fresh strawberries picked from the garden, a new dress, or a baseball game with the neighborhood kids. Would you have thought of that memory right this minute had I not asked you to? Not likely. It takes someone or something else to trigger moments in our memory.

My next question is…Are you thinking about the whole day or are you thinking about the moment? The moment. Our memory is made up of moments. People with dementia have these moments in their memory just like you and I, but they can't pull a moment out of the darkness. Not until they *see* a swing, *smell* the bread, *taste* a strawberry, or *feel* a baseball glove will the memory be triggered.

Before we can create moments of joy, we need to understand the person with Alzheimer's…**understand** that they lose their short-term memory. How do we know they lose their short-term memory? They repeat the same question over and over and over again. And if you ask them, "What did you have for breakfast?," they will answer something like, "I don't know. I didn't get any." What if you ask them about the family reunion they went to last weekend? Their response will likely be, "What family reunion? I haven't seen my family in months."

Even though they lose their short-term memory, they can retain long-term memory as the disease progresses. Whose responsibility is it to chat about their long term memories *instead of* their short-term memories? Ours. Instead of asking, "What did you have for breakfast?," or "Did you have a good visit with your son last night?," chat about the memories that are ingrained in them: "You love bacon and eggs." "Your son has big brown eyes, just like you."

One of my joys is walking in the rain. I was out walking in the rain one night and decided to stop by the nursing home to create a moment of joy. A lady came up to me and said, "Honey you are so wet, can I get you a towel?" I responded, "I love walking in the rain. I am a water girl, and a really good swimmer." She piped back, "I'm a good swimmer! When I was eight years old there was two kids in the river and they didn't look like they were going to make it. I jumped in, grabbed the girl by the hair, told that boy he better hang on, and I swam. I could not touch the bottom. But then I did touch the bottom and pushed those kids to shore." I gasped, "You saved their lives?!?" She answered, "Honey, all I know is I was shaking and I didn't swim for two years."

How many times do you think I heard that story in the fifteen minutes we were chatting? At least five. What triggered her story? My hair was wet. You too will hear from someone a story over and over again. You have a choice…"Ugh, if I have to hear *that* story one more time!" Or you can think, "I'd better remember this story for this person." Because as the disease progresses she will lose the ability to communicate her story. When that happens, what do you think will create joy for her? Us telling her her story.

I wish I could hear the story my mom told me over and over. It is the very thing I miss now that she is no longer living. —A DAUGHTER

That story that irritates you may be the very thing that creates joy. In fact, two months later while I was visiting that community I walked up to that lady and said, "Have you been swimming lately?" She answered, "No, but when I was eight years old there was two kids in the river and they didn't look like they were going to make it…" She told me the whole story all over again. What did I have to say to trigger her story? *Swimming.* Imagine if everyone knew to use the word *swimming* with this lady—if every visitor, every caregiver went up to her and said, "Hey, have you been swimming lately?" Then she would get to tell her story over and over. Would she have a better day? Absolutely! Because telling her story leaves her with a good feeling. A good feeling about saving those kids.

This next part is a little more confusing: As the disease progresses, they get younger in their mind. In other words, they lose more and more short-term memory. We know this because who do they ask for? Their parents, *who are deceased,* their spouse, their kids. But when her husband is in the room she is thinking, "Ew, I will be nice to that man for about ten minutes but then he has to go." She is looking for her young, handsome beau. Or they will wonder, "Where are my kids?" But when their kids come to visit they do not recognize them because they are looking for their *little* kids.

Figure out what age they are living in their mind because this is where their memories are. If she is constantly looking for her mom, how old do you think she is at this moment? Probably adolescent. If she's constantly looking for her husband but doesn't recognize him, she is in her twenties or thirties. If she is constantly looking for her kids but doesn't recognize them, what age are her kids in her mind? Four? Seven?

Our whole goal is to help them *feel* like whoever they're looking for is perfectly okay in this moment. If they're looking for their mom, how do we make them feel like their mom is okay? Where would their mom be? At home? But if you say their mom is at home, then you trigger them to want to go home. Take the word "home" *out* of your vocabulary. It's better to say, "Your mom will be right back," or "Your mom is in the kitchen." Where would her husband be? At work? In the field? Fishing?

People think this is lying because: "Their mom is no longer living. She is not in the kitchen." "Their husband is no longer living. He is not in the field." Go ahead, give it your best shot and tell the person *your truth.* Tell the person their husband is no longer living. How does that make them *feel* in this moment? *Confused, distraught, anxious, and alone.* How do they function when they feel these emotions? Consider they can't function. Who suffers the repercussions when they feel angry, sad, alone, scared? *We do.* Do they change when you tell them their husband is no longer living? Do they say, "Oh yeah, that's right," and never ask you the question again? No. They cannot change. This is a disease. They are doing the best that they can with the memories they have left. They are not asking these questions just to irritate you. Who is the only one who can change? You are.

It was obvious a caregiver didn't live Evelyn's truth because she came into my office upset because her mom had died, her husband had died, and she couldn't get to their funerals, both of which she thought were being held in this building. We walked for a bit and chatted. I knew she was Christian, so we went back to my office, sang hymns, and prayed. When she left she told me how much she enjoyed church and that she hadn't been to a church service in such a long time. These simple moments brought her to a peaceful place.

—RAELEEN BOYKIN

While I was visiting a community, a lady in distress asked me, "Have you seen my sister?" I responded as I normally do: "Yes, I have. She said she's looking forward to visiting you." She replied, "Oh thank God…because that lady over there said she was dead. I need to sit down. I am not feeling so well."

People will have literal pain because of the answers we give them. *Live in their truth.* Make them *feel* that whomever they are looking for is perfectly okay right now. Remember…short-term memory loss: you get to keep changing your answer until you find the one that works.

Families also tend to focus on who this person was in the recent past. Dad was a businessman. Dad was a board member. Dad was an accountant. But when we meet him, all he wants is Betsy. "Betsy! Betsy! Betsy!" Who could Betsy be, based on what his kids have told us? His wife? His secretary? His child? Betsy could be just about anybody. Who has to figure out who Betsy is? We do. Because how many times does he look for her throughout day? Over and over.

We think Betsy is his wife, and we say to him, "She is uptown getting her hair done." Then he looks like, "Liar, crazy woman!" Can you not tell when you give someone the wrong answer? They look at you like, "Where did you fall from?" Because…for this person, Betsy was his cow. "Betsy's uptown getting her hair done?!?" What?!? This is the only disease where you get to keep changing your answer every thirty seconds until you find the one that works.

When you finally figure out Betsy is the cow, can you say to him, "You don't have a cow. You are eighty-two years old"? No, because now he will be worried about the cow. Where would Betsy be to be perfectly okay? "She's in the barn," "She's out in the back forty," or "I just milked her." Again, your whole goal is to make them feel like whoever they want or whatever they are looking for is perfectly okay in this moment. How old is he in his mind if he is looking for Betsy? Maybe fifteen or sixteen. If he is fifteen in his mind, whose responsibility is it to chat about his siblings and grandparents *instead of* the grandkids that visited yesterday? Ours.

Let's say that in their mind they are in their twenties, and at that time they lived in Missouri, but now they live in Arizona. In this moment where do they believe they are living? Missouri. Who has to Google their hometown in Missouri or get a map of Missouri? We do.

They may even revert back to their native language. If the person lived in Germany until he was fifteen, he may start speaking German again, which means you may have to learn a few German words. If you sing a simple song such as *Happy Birthday*, the *ABCs*, or the *1-2-3s*, it may trigger the person to speak English again.

At some point they will no longer recognize themselves, so when they talk to the mirror they are really talking to someone else. That person in the mirror is much older than they are. Talking to a mirror may have a negative effect because the person in the mirror doesn't talk back or looks ill. If that's the case, remove the mirror. But if they are having a lovely conversation with the person in the mirror, let it go.

Once we realize what age they are living in their mind at this moment, then we will be more likely to connect with them and possibly find out things we never knew before. (*Note:* The age at which they think they are living shifts throughout the day. In the morning they may be more lucid, but in the evening they may be looking for their mom. Having this understanding is like having a window into a person's mind. And we are here to bring light into that window.)

People ask me, "How do I know if I have found the right answer?" Just look at the person's face. It will tell you everything. And if it works, it works. Don't question it, no matter how bizarre the answer seems to you. Your goal is to create a better reaction. You're not shooting for a perfect reaction, just a better reaction. When you find the answer that works to the question they ask fifty times a day, tell everyone!!! It is a treasure that will surely create a better day.

Our value lies in what we are and what we have been, not in our ability to recite the recent past. —HOMER, A MAN WITH ALZHEIMER'S

Newfound Understanding

To Let Go Takes Love

To "let go" does not mean stop caring;
it means I can't do it for someone else.
To "let go" is not to cut myself off;
it's to realize that I can't control another.
To "let go" is to admit to powerlessness,
which means the outcome is not in my hands.
To "let go" is to try not to change or blame another;
I can only change myself.
To "let go" is not to "care for," but to "care about."
To "let go" is not to fix, but to be supportive.
To "let go" is not to judge,
but to allow another to be a human being.
To "let go" is not to deny, but to accept.
To "let go" is not to nag, scold, or argue,
but instead to search out my own shortcomings and correct them.
To "let go" is not to adjust everything to my desires,
but to take each day as it comes, and to cherish myself in it.
To "let go" is not to regret the past,
but to grow and live for the future.
To "let go" is to fear less and love more.

—ROBERT PAUL GILLES

Family Moments

Love and care with a genuine heart. —Jolene

I Promised...

Sometimes out of fear we ask loved ones to promise things we shouldn't. And sometimes out of love we make promises we just can't keep. When we really love someone, it means trusting them to do what is right. When we exact a promise from our loved ones, like, "Promise me you'll never put me in a nursing home," or "Promise me you'll never let me get *that* way," we are asking for promises that cannot be kept.

When we marry someone we promise to love, honor, and protect them in sickness and in health—until death. There are different ways to fulfill that promise. You promise to be their spouse, not their caregiver. Sometimes being a caregiver is beyond your capability, which means the most loving thing to do would be to let someone else be the caregiver. When you are married, doing what is honorable, what is right, means doing what is honorable and right for both of you. If you decide to be the caregiver, but then there comes a point at which you just cannot mentally or physically do it anymore, then the honorable and right thing to do for both of you is to let someone else give care.

If you have decided to caregive, ask yourself these tough questions: "Why did I choose to caregive? Out of obligation? Promise? Because I am the only child without kids to take care of? Or is it because caregiving is what I want to do?" Caregiving based on obligation or promise often creates resentment and/or guilt. To sustain yourself emotionally you must *want* to do it. And even if caregiving is something you want to do, allow yourself to reevaluate along the way to make sure it is something you want to continue to do.

As a caregiver you need help. Research shows that if you try to do it all by yourself, there is a good chance you will end up in the hospital, or pass away *before* the person with Alzheimer's does. Do you

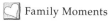

really think the person you are caring for would want you to lose your health, or your life, in the process of caring for them? People have great compassion for the person afflicted with Alzheimer's because they can see what is happening to them. But most often the caregiver's suffering remains unnoticed. Take note of the caregiver's well-being because they are important too.

Someday you'll need someone to take care of you. Please don't leave the decision about how to take care of you up to your kids. Kids rarely agree, and this could end in conflict. I urge you to give your spouse and children permission NOT to take care of you. I have met so many individuals still harboring guilty feelings all because they made a promise they couldn't keep. And they continue to carry this guilt around even after the person is gone.

While still of sound mind, set forth in a living will how you would prefer to live the last part of your journey on this earth. Be sure they are realistic wishes and clearly communicate them to all involved. This is a gift you can give now.

On our fifty-seventh wedding anniversary we ate our lunch together. My wife remarked that we did not have children. Then she said, "We have been married for a long time, and that has given me more time to love you." I laughed and time stood still while I caught my breath. It may be awhile before I again experience such a moment of joy.

—DON ALEXANDER, HUSBAND AND CAREGIVER

Even after all this time the Sun never says to the Earth you owe me. —HAFIZ, PERSIAN POET OF THE 1300s

Newfound UnPromise

"I Can't Leave 'Em"

Written by an individual affected by Alzheimer's.

"I'm sorry, we just can't attend the graduation because John ..."

"I can't stay. I have to get home to my wife."

"Thanks for the invite, but I just can't."

"Sweetheart, I'm not going to be able to make it to your wedding."

"We can't make it to Robbie's basketball game. It's not a good day."

Do any of these statements sound familiar to you? What do they reflect? A caregiver whose world has shrunken down to virtually their own home, or their relationship to just the person they are caring for? When is enough, enough? What are the markers that tell us the situation needs to change, that a decision has to be made? Must we keep going until we ourselves are in need of antidepressants or antianxiety medication just to cope? To what extent are we obligated to carry on as is?

Ah, that's the key word: *obligated.* To understand how far we are obligated to go, we must first determine what our obligations are. Look at the numbered rings on the next page. List your obligations on the lines: #1 being the most important, #2 being the next important, and so on.

What did you list as your #1 obligation? Yourself? Your children or spouse? To be happy? The center circle is your *core obligation.* It is who you are. It's the primary obligation that supersedes all others, and to violate it is to violate what makes you, you. If you believe in a Supreme Being (or Beings), then that may be your core obligation. Or maybe it's your principles (honesty, loyalty, patience, etc.). Human beings, emotional states, or material objects wouldn't be your core obligation. That place alone is reserved for your principles (which make us human), or for God (from whom you derive your principles).

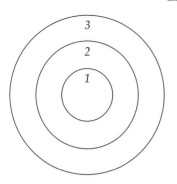

What does all of this mean? As a caregiver, the person you are caring for is more than likely #2 or #3 on your rings of obligation. If you aren't violating your core obligation when caring for them, then you're right in what you're doing. But what if it comes to a point where you can no longer be kind, patient, and loving with them? Or with others? Or yourself? Then you are violating your #1 (core) obligation, and it's time for a change.

> *My brother came to visit me. My husband has Alzheimer's and I was obviously showing frustration, anger, and resentment toward my husband. My brother looked at me and gave me advice that saved my life: "Let someone else take care of him for awhile. Don't wait until your love turns to hate."*
>
> —A WIFE

Oftentimes when a person is at their wit's end, they will exclaim in exasperation, "I just want to do what's right!" Okay then, look to your core obligation for guidance. It is this compass that points you in the right direction. Without it we are lost.

Remember, your core obligation is who you are. Don't lose yourself in the midst of this journey.

Learn character from trees, value from roots and change from leaves. —TASNEEM HAMEED

Newfound Core

Love:
Noun or Verb

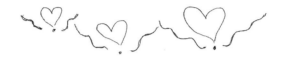

Phone call between two brothers:

Steve: "Ryan and I went to Mom and Dad's last weekend."

Dave: "Oh yeah, how was Dad doing?"

Steve: "Much worse. When Ryan threw a pop can in the trash, Dad jumped up and got all mad, saying he was wasting five cents. And when Ryan opened the blinds to let some light in, Dad overreacted terribly. It made Ryan all upset. I won't be taking him over there anymore."

Dave: "Ryan is fifteen years old now. Don't you think he should be learning to deal with difficult things in life?"

If you look up the word *love* in the dictionary, you see that it can be a noun or it can be a verb. A verb implies action, which is the kind of love needed in difficult circumstances—love in action. But unfortunately for most people love follows that old maxim, "When all is said and done, more will have been said than done."

Consider this: Your father has Alzheimer's and your mother is caring for him. When you go over there he doesn't remember your name; he gets upset over nonsensical things, makes weird noises at the dinner table, and says things you can't comprehend. You are embarrassed for him and unsettled when you leave.

Time goes by and you haven't gone back to see your parents. You tell yourself, and your mother who is asking, that work has you tied up, or that your kids' activities don't give you any time to go home to visit. It's always "something," but it's never really the truth, which is that you don't want to see your dad that way—that you don't want to deal with it. So you keep making up excuses not to visit, and feeling miserable about that, and in the process making your mother miserable too.

You are a master practitioner of "noun love," the do-nothing love. You prefer to love from afar where it's easy and takes little effort. You try to ease your guilt by telling yourself that your mother has it handled, or that your siblings or the neighbors are there helping them. But you never actually verify any of that because deep down you really don't want to find out that pretty much everyone else has also abandoned them.

Perhaps you should reflect a bit on who changed your dirty diapers, wiped your runny nose, picked you up when you fell down, and taught you the ABC's, how to tie your shoes, and how to ride a bike. Or how about just the basics that they fed, clothed, and loved you. All of those things are "verb love"—action love—and yet here you are repaying them with noun love?

What kind of love do you want to teach your children? How can they learn to be loving, caring, compassionate adults if you do not show them through your own actions? To love others when it is easy, and even more so when it is hard. To go where others do not, stay when others leave, and leave only when it's loving to do so. If we live a life of love like this, it will truly be a life worth living, and a light shining in the darkness to others.

This diagnosis has actually brought us closer together. There is somewhat of a role reversal; I have taken over the mothering role and that's alright with me. Mom has made so many sacrifices in her life for me. Now it's my turn. She will always be my mother and I love her dearly. —A DAUGHTER

A High Practice: To Love ourselves and others in our humanness. —SISTER JENNY, S.P.

Newfound Loving Action

Taking Care of Yourself

Just as we need to find out what relieves stress for a person with dementia, we need to find what relieves stress for us.

Walking, napping, a hot lavender bath, getting a massage, getting your hair done, playing cards with friends, going uptown for coffee...alone. If you haven't already, please add water, water, water. Hot water with lemon "cleans out the pipes," so an older man told me. A spoonful of peanut butter before bed helps you sleep, so said Flossy.

Whenever I meet healthy older people, I ask, "What's your secret?" One man said peanut butter on saltine crackers every morning, and a ninety-four-year-old said a martini every night. It seems to me you gotta find your own tricks because there is no rhyme or reason. Whatever calms *you* down and relaxes *your* body...do that. On the flip side, it's just as important to pay attention to what drains you and avoid those situations and people at all costs. When someone calls to give you their opinion, simply excuse yourself by saying, "I have to use the bathroom," and hang up. You do not have the energy to appease others.

Of most importance is to take time off from caregiving—at least two days a week. I have heard an infinite number of excuses for why caregivers can't take care of themselves. Who is the only one who can give you permission to take care of you? *You.* Ask for help, and be *clear* about how others can help.

If your best friend told you, "My spouse isn't sleeping at night. He walked out the front door, walked two blocks, and didn't know how to get back. He didn't know who I was the other day and yelled at me to get out of his house." What advice would you give your best friend? To get help? If these things are happening, be your best friend. Take your advice. It may be time to get help.

I strongly recommend getting involved in a support group. I know that feels like one more thing, but when you meet another spouse who has already been through the journey, they will help you more than this book will. When you meet another daughter, she can give you emotional wisdom I cannot give you.

Open the door and share your story. You will be surprised at how many others have a similar story. Simply knowing you're not alone on this journey is priceless. If the support group drains you, find another, or just meet someone for coffee.

I met two women who were both taking care of their moms. One took the ladies (moms) every Monday/Wednesday and the other took the ladies every Tuesday/Thursday. Brilliant.

I can make this journey sound like butterflies and cupcakes. However, that cannot be further from the true suffering and pain that is caused by Alzheimer's. But you are on this road, and you want to get to your destination as safely as possible. Watch for signs moment by moment to give yourself direction. Pull off the road, take a catnap whenever possible, and accept help from others when something breaks down. In fact, take a couple of friends with you so they can drive when you get worn out.

Just start with one thing that makes you feel better. Many days will end in exhaustion and you probably won't even have the energy to ask for help. Your body is your compass. It will tell you before your mind does when enough is enough. Pause and listen. Listen to what your body, mind, and soul are telling you.

No one should have to lose both of their parents to Alzheimer's. Take care of yourself too. —Words of Wisdom

---

Newfound Calm

"They Look Great!"

Your brother calls long distance and has a perfectly wonderful conversation with Dad. He tells you, "Dad sounds really good. Do you think we can move him back home?" The neighbor stops by and has a lovely visit. Upon leaving he says, "He looks really good. You must be doing alright."

How does it make you, the caregiver, feel when others think it's not that bad…Resentful? Unsupported? Like you're the one going crazy or that you're doing something wrong to have created all of this?

Your brother is having a wonderful conversation with Dad over the phone because Dad recognizes his voice (and isn't confused by seeing his face), and the telephone triggers a social response. We can be yelling at someone in one moment, but when the phone rings or someone knocks on the door our disposition changes instantly. The person with Alzheimer's does the same thing. They can look physically well and act perfectly fine for a moment, but underneath they are lost.

When anyone says, "It's not that bad," simply tell them that you need a break and ask if they would like to come take care of the person for a few days. It will only take a few hours. When they experience first-hand what you have been experiencing, then and only then will they believe something is wrong. But you, as the caregiver, must leave the premises because the person with Alzheimer's will act fine as long as they see you, because they feel safe with you. Go to a hotel or a friend's house. Within hours your brother will ask you to come home because there is something "wrong" and he needs to get back to work.

Anyone who disagrees with how you are giving care, let them know, "Dad can come live with you." The only one who holds the truth is the one who gives the care. Everyone else just holds an opinion.

As a caregiver, write down ten ways in which others can help. People want to help—they just don't know how. As a family, identify in what way each family member or friend is gifted. The person who is good with numbers handles the finances. The person who likes to be on the computer can research care communities to prepare for the day when the person needs more care. The favorite grandchild can take Grandma out to eat or for a country drive to give the caregiver regular breaks. The most responsible person can set up appointments and stay on top of meds and schedules. We are all gifted in different areas. Be clear about "how you need help" so that others can help in a way that lightens the load.

My brothers were more likely to help when I was specific. I didn't attack the whole situation, just what I needed right now. I said to one brother, "I would like to go out to eat with a friend. Do you think you could come over for a couple of hours?" To my other brother, who likes to go out to eat, I simply said, "Dad is hungry. Will you take him out to eat?"

All you know is what you think you know, but that isn't always what's real. —CARRIE VAUGHN

Newfound Support

Helping Hands

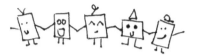

Caregivers will need the help of others to get through this. They are on call 24/7 in their hearts, if not literally. They feel a deep, personal burden about the needs they expect themselves to fulfill. So a helping hand might not be accepted...

> *The caregiver:* "No, you don't have to do this."
> *Your response:* "Yes, I want to."
> *The caregiver:* "No, I've never left him before."
> *Your response:* "Just go. We will be fine."
> *The caregiver:* "He might..."
> *Your response:* "You don't have to worry. I got it."
> *The caregiver:* "Well..."
> *Your response:* "We will be just fine. Enjoy yourself."
> *The caregiver:* "Are you sure?"
> *Your response:* "Yes, I'm sure. Take as long as you like."
> *The caregiver:* "I don't know."
> *Your response:* "Well I do. Now scoot" (with a smile).
> The caregiver hesitates... *Your response:* "Scoot."

Once the caregiver experiences that it is okay for someone else to help, they will be quicker to accept help the next time. The first time is the most difficult.

Caregivers are exhausted and don't have the energy to ask for help or even figure out how others can help. Keep it simple. Ask the caregiver what are five ways we can help, and get them to be specific. It's important for someone to set up a help schedule. When we visit or help all at once, we are actually adding more stress.

How to give a helping hand

* Do their laundry
* Schedule people to drop off food every other day
* Mow their lawn (Don't ask them, just do it)
* Ask what you can pick up at the grocery store
* Take the person with dementia on a country drive or to a ball game so the caregiver can have a "me" break
* Offer to stay with the person so the caregiver can run errands, get their hair done, or visit a friend
* Give them meals to put in the freezer
* Mail movie tickets or restaurant certificates anonymously
* Clean their house and do dishes with them
* Share your garden vegetables: "I have too many…"
* Stay overnight so the caregiver can fully rest

Whatever might ease their journey…do that. Sometimes it's better when the caregiver is out of the house. It's too easy for them to feel guilty if they are watching you help. And when helping, reassure them by saying, "You are my friend. I care about you, so please let me help."

Pair up in threes. —Yogi Berra

Newfound Help

"I'm Here to Take Care of You!"

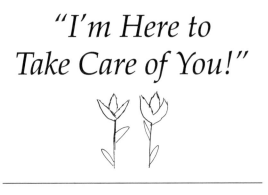

The person with dementia truly doesn't believe there is anything wrong with them or that they need help. So if you are there to take care of them don't be surprised when they ask you to leave and slam the door behind you. It's better if they feel like you stopped by as a friend, or someone who needs their help.

> "Hi, my name is Billy. I am Pat's son. He told me you had a '56 Chevy in the garage. I would love to see it."
> "My mom says you make an amazing cherry pie. Would you teach me how to make one?"
> "I missed the bus. I'm kind of stuck."
> "My car broke down. Any chance I can wait here until it gets fixed?"

If older grandchildren want to earn extra money, try: "Mom, Alicia doesn't get her apartment for another week. It would really be a blessing to her to have a place to stay." (Another week, another week, another week…) If you are a single mom, bring your child with you and say: "Suzi wanted to visit you today." Another option is to introduce the caregiver as your friend, then fake a phone call and say: "I have to go to work. Do you mind if Justin stays here until I get back?"

You might think you have to hire a "professional" to take care of them. But I think you would be better off hiring a bartender, a beautician, a teenager, a single mom, a church lady, or a retired man. Hire the social person, the extrovert, the one who chats with complete strangers wherever they go. It doesn't matter their age or experience…what matters is their ability to "be liked" instantly.

If they don't like you and want you to leave, do so. Go outside, change into a different outfit (backpack 'n' pigtails) and come back as a kid who just got off the school bus and is waiting for your mom to

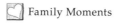

pick you up. Or simply say, "Okay" and go into another room where they cannot see you. It can be incredibly uncomfortable for the person to even sit in a room knowing that a caregiver is there to watch them.

Be someone who goes to the same church, or someone who knows their daughter, or someone they would want to invite in for coffee. This way it's about them being the hostess and taking care of you.

> Instead of putting others in their place put yourself in their place. —AMISH PROVERB

Newfound Friend

"You Can't Drive"

When you say to the person, "You can't drive," do they like you? Absolutely not. Instead, get ten sets of car keys and scatter them around the house. Trying each set of keys is exercise, and you hold onto the keys that work.

Please do not sell the car. Even if you agreed to sell the car, in two weeks they won't remember. Every time they look in the driveway and don't see the car, how does it make them feel? Angry and upset. Go ahead, try to reason with someone who has short-term memory loss. "Remember…we sold the car." You can't get someone to remember, who can't remember.

A daughter was visiting her mom and her mom accused her of selling the car. She didn't sell her car—her brother did—but her mom blamed her. My response to anyone in this situation: Tell your mom you are sorry and ask for forgiveness.

A better option is to let a grandchild use the car so you still have it. "Johnny needed the car to run errands." If they don't like that answer, then say, "Okay, I will call him and get it back." In that moment, they have the hope of getting it back. But you aren't really getting it back. If it's a person who won't settle until they get it back, then by all means get it back, but disable it. For a woman that often means simply taking out the battery, but a man will have the battery replaced in ten minutes.

A mechanic, whose dad was a mechanic and had Alzheimer's, shared this solution: "It wasn't until I replaced the coil wire with a vacuum line or a small black suction tube that he could not fix the car. For vehicles built after 2000, remove the fuel pump fuse because it will act like it is out of gas but the fuel gage will show it's full."

* *Have the doctor write a note saying they can no longer drive.*
* *Replace the car with a golf cart.*
* *Get a new car because they can't figure out new things.*
* *Call the D.O.T. and tell them you would like the person to take the test but simply receive an identification card.*
* *Say, "We don't have insurance right now."*
* *Say, "Sweetheart, you have driven all these years. It's my turn."*

We live in a rural community. I let my husband get in the truck and then I called the cops. When he got home he was mad at the cops, not at me, for taking his keys.

With my mom, I tell her it is a rental car and the insurance only covers me.

Unfortunately, families will wait and wait and wait for permission. This person will not likely say, "Hey, here are my keys. I shouldn't be driving." It just won't happen that way. What will happen:

* The person will stop in the middle of an intersection and think they are stopping in a parking lot.
* The person will drive for six hours lost and think they have been driving for thirty minutes.
* The person will think they hit a bump, when instead they hit a pedestrian.
* The person will get lost on a route they have taken a hundred times before.

I was going through an intersection when out of nowhere a car slammed into my front passenger side. I was hit so hard my car was now facing the other direction. As I sat there shaking in shock, I watched the car that hit me swerve all over the neighboring yards and continue on for another four blocks. The car did not stop until it hit the front step of a house. I came to find out the driver was a ninety-three-year-old man with dementia. He had mistaken the gas pedal for the brake. It was very lucky that no one got hurt. The outcome could have been devastating.

This decision is one of the most difficult you will make because driving is something they have been doing for a lifetime. They don't realize their judgment is impaired. The truth is found by driving *with* a person.

I, as a person who is supposedly an expert on Alzheimer's, have struggled to practice what I preach. I have an older friend whom I love dearly, and one night she drove us home. She frequently crossed over the middle line and swerved toward the edge. It was a white-knuckle ride for me. This beautiful, independent woman has traveled the world and now has difficulty driving home in the dark. I spoke with my girlfriends about how she shouldn't be driving, but we didn't take her keys. I have not been able to do what I am asking my readers to do. Much, much, much easier said than done. —JOLENE

In some places there are people whose job it is to drive with others to determine if they are capable of driving. It may be easier for you and me if a stranger informs them they can't drive. Then, as a friend you can be there to let them vent, and together as a group of friends you can "pick them up."

Or, have a neighbor man put on a police uniform and take away his keys or driver's license. A man is going to be more cooperative with a big man in a uniform and you don't have to get the law involved. For big guys out there this can be a whole new business venture, a full-time job, simply helping us ladies with our men.

This concept also applies to someone who has always owned a gun. If you remove the gun, they won't forget about it. They will only be angry because they can't find it. Keep the gun, but disable it. This doesn't mean simply hiding the bullets because they will find a way to replace them. It means to make their gun look like it works, but it absolutely does not work.

A son was visiting his dad. They were arguing, and the dad in that moment didn't recognize "his boy." No one will ever really know what all happened between the two men, but unfortunately the dad shot his boy, whom he obviously saw as a threatening man.

Do not wait—Do not wait—Do not wait for permission. At some point it becomes no choice. If you can't do it, ask someone who can. (Any man in full uniform can pretend to be the authority we need to calm him down.)

Drive carefully. It's not only cars that can be recalled by their maker. —Unknown

Newfound Transportation

Finances

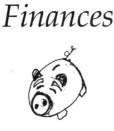

This is a very complicated subject and is best addressed when this person is cognitively able to make sound decisions. Make sure the right thing is done for this person, and that the money they have worked hard to earn is being used as they wish.

Every week I took this lady out to eat, to buy treats from the bakery, to go to the symphony, and to get her hair done. Her money was used to take care of her wants and wishes. —Sister Richard, S.P.

While this person is cognitively able, have them choose someone they trust to become their power of attorney. The person chosen must be able to make hard decisions. While they are still at home, bring everyone involved together so that wants and wishes are established. (Holding conversations together is imperative, and maybe even record them.) If there are significant assets, an attorney should be present.

If there are no children involved, whose role is it? Decide while you are able.

I stepped into a situation where I could clearly see that an elder, Helen, was about to be taken advantage of for her considerable savings. We discussed the situation and I presented an option of having a bank trust department handle her cash and assets. She didn't have any reliable family members left who were willing or able; she only had an old neighbor who had drained her sister's assets to the degree that there was no money left to take care of her needs. Helen readily agreed, and the trust officer really listened to her, treated her well, and conserved her money through her passing.

Once we had her financial business taken care of, it was important to know that her long-term health care would be in good hands. She had no one, so I volunteered. This was one of the most heart-wrenching things I've ever done. I didn't know her well, and she had already started to show signs of dementia. I worked with her while she was still able and learned her wishes. I was her health care decision maker for over six years, and multiple times I was required to make difficult decisions. The final decision I made was to discontinue treatment, which ultimately led to her death. Those decisions still weigh heavily. —Linda

Health and well-being are more important than money. Often adult children disagree about how money should be handled. I have seen children who are financially drowning because they don't want to use their parent's money. Then there are those who won't move their parent into assisted living because they are dependent on the income from the parent's care. I have also experienced siblings who wouldn't allow another sibling to use their parent's money unless they produce a receipt. Ugh! —Natalie

You can give the person the illusion of control by letting them sign a few checks, but pay most bills online. Or ask the bank to provide checks that require two signatures, then if one slips by it isn't valid.

My friend with Alzheimer's was living alone and would pay bills twice or not at all. She resisted the transition to online banking because she didn't want to change her system. I had to reassure her over and over that after this is set up she wouldn't even need to think about it. Eventually, most of her bills were set up on automatic withdrawal. She still wanted to physically write the check to pay for her rent and walk it to her landlord, so I let that one go. One of the two most important things we did was to transfer $400 of spending money every month onto a bankcard for gas, groceries, and whatever. The bankcard looked just like her original card. That way when she was out of money it wouldn't let her go in the hole, which had been a constant problem. She would overspend her account, and then the bank would charge her $15 every day she was over the limit. So every month she was giving the bank $200 to $300.

The other best thing we did was to have her brother pay her monthly bill for her secondary health insurance. There were times she did not pay, and her health insurance was canceled. Then her health bills were not covered and they piled up. It was very overwhelming. So her brother pays that bill every month on time and that got rid of some worries. She seems to be able to manage life doing it this way for now. We will cross our fingers. —Karen, a friend

From STEVEN K. FREEL, CLU, ChFC, CFP, Vision Financial Group

- Goals keep you safe—keep your money safe. People over sixty-five are most likely to be taken advantage of financially.
- Make sure the power of attorney for property (business) is up to date and has at least three people named in order to serve. Make sure they understand they have a fiduciary position.
- Someone will be taking care of all this after you are gone. Wouldn't it be better to talk about it to make sure your wishes are understood?
- Review all ownership and beneficiary data on assets to make sure they are correct.
- Do everything that needs to be done sooner rather than later.
- Bring in a financial planner, CFP, or attorney to offer third-party advice. It needs to be a real planner—not a sales person. It's better for a professional to suggest than a family.
- You may have it all taken care of so why not get a second opinion. Two things will happen:
  - There will still be time to fix a problem if needed.
  - You'll have peace of mind that all is good.
- We are family. You took care of me financially when I needed and I am very grateful. Let me repay that and pass on the same blessing. Who really gets more—the giver or the receiver?
- Make a long-term plan: five to ten years of how and where to access money to pay for care. Which assets are used first, second, and so forth. What are the tax consequences? At what point is Medicaid an option? Understand the guidelines in your state.
- Understand that all this will take time and emotional energy; everyone underestimates how much. Non-caregiver family members need to compensate caregivers. Have a plan for how to do it and the cost so there's no misunderstanding later.

In general, older people worry constantly about money, especially if in their mind they have reverted back to a time when they didn't have any. They may have more than enough money in the bank to pay for everything, but a verbal reassurance is not enough. Print out their bank statement so they can carry it in their wallet or purse, or create a fake bank statement with an extra $20,000 to create a moment of joy.

My dad used to always keep a hundred dollar bill in his pocket. I asked him about that today and told him that that could always get you out of trouble. He looked at me and smiled...then said it could always get you into trouble, too.   —CHUCK

Money doesn't solve all problems, but it could solve the money problems. —UNKNOWN

Newfound Investment

Funerals

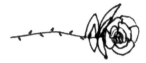

(*Should we take them?*)

No one can predict how someone will respond at a funeral. There are so many factors to consider. What stage of Alzheimer's are they in? If in an early stage, then it may be good to take them because it allows the person the opportunity to grieve, but it does not mean they will remember that someone they love has died. If they do remember, it may be in distorted fragments. Middle stages? I don't know. There is a place for an action that contributes to the greater good: If the person attends the funeral, the entire family will feel better knowing they were there. But we must be aware of whose wants we are fulfilling. Late stages? No, in my opinion, because taking them out of their familiar environment and adding the stress of being around so many people is too much. Whom does it benefit? Instead, have a quiet moment in this person's room to celebrate whomever has passed on. Bring old pictures, memorabilia, and things that trigger memories. You can laugh, cry, and hold one another during this time. It's not about getting the person to remember who died, but remembering who lived.

In care communities I do think it's important that there is some sort of visual gesture to let everyone know when a person has passed on. Instead of shuttling a person's body out the back door, create an honoring, a ritual, and escort the body past everyone. Maybe there's a certain quilt you use to cover the body, or a pastor or priest who always presides over the bodies of those who have passed. Something special that signifies something important and sacred has occurred. Later in the day, with everyone, take time to celebrate this person; give residents and caregivers the opportunity to honor and express all that shows up.

Simply create the space to allow all the feelings when someone goes "home."

Wisdom growing in wounded places, seasons of sorrow in the soil of suffering. —DONNA BUTLER, S.P.

Newfound Remembrance

Outings with Less Stress

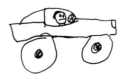

Before you take them out, sit and visit for a bit to get reacquainted. Because of short-term memory loss, you may be a stranger in this moment and they may be nervous about leaving with you—even if you had a nice long visit yesterday.

> *My wife tried to jump out of the car. She didn't know who I was and where I was taking her, so in that moment she didn't feel safe with me.*

> *A lady with Alzheimer's asked when walking with a man she should have known, "Who are you?" He tried to tell her he was her friend. Then she simply said, "You have no idea how scary this is."*

Keep outings simple: Take a short drive in the country, visit a friend, watch children play at the park, feed the ducks, or go for a walk in a quiet neighborhood. Always bring a sack lunch or a bag of goodies to nibble on. Avoid eating at restaurants, especially during prime hours. If you really want to go out to eat, go during off hours and ask for a private room away from the noise and rush. Avoid malls and zoos, or anyplace with too much stimulation.

> *A woman approached me wondering whether it was still a good idea to take her dad out to breakfast. "How is he?," I asked. She responded that he was very quiet. I then asked her if he had always been quiet. "No," she replied. I told her that she might instead consider bringing breakfast to him to see if he has a better reaction. He was her teacher.*

The person may seem to enjoy the excursion, but the real proof is how they are when they get home. It may take two days or two weeks to recover from one outing.

A family brought their mom back to the community after a drive. She would not go inside—she wanted to go home. They insisted that this was her home, and even tried to force her. This little gray-haired lady, weighing only one hundred pounds, won the battle. A third person came along and nonchalantly said, "Your daughters are inside waiting to eat lunch with you. Are you hungry?" She said yes then walked back in. It was that easy. Unfortunately the family is now afraid to take their mother on another outing.

Like anyone else, they have good days and bad days. Pay attention to their emotional reactions. If they are confused or anxious, you know you will have to cut the trip short or just stay home.

My mother-in-law insisted every day that she wanted to go see her relatives in Oregon, which was ten hours away. So I said, "Today is the day. Pack your lunch—we are going to see your relatives." I drove a half hour to relatives living in the next town, and then another half hour to other relatives. When we got home in the evening, she was perfectly content and tired. She said, "That was a lovely trip."

We took my dad on a trip to go see his sister. Our intention was good but my dad dropped into another level of dementia. He thought he was again in the Vietnam war, and we couldn't console him. My suggestion to everyone: Skype or call instead of taking the trip.

To let scenery become your playground, grocerer, and bed womb is to know true nourishment. —MICHAEL BILLINGTON

Newfound Outing

Holidays 'n'
Family Reunions

Holidays and family reunions are very stressful for a person with dementia. Not only do we take them out of their familiar environment, but we also invite everyone over and ask the person to be "normal" again. The kids think, "Mom should be there." Could it be that we inflict our own values and standards on people with dementia?

The person will be nice and act perfectly fine for a short while, but eventually due to utter confusion they will say, "I want to go home." Or they have an unexpected outburst, which essentially means, "I can't handle this situation." Family gatherings are actually the time when everyone gets to experience firsthand that something is wrong, which is a blessing in disguise because awareness is the key to doing it differently.

We had Thanksgiving at our house again this year. Late afternoon my husband looked at me and said, "Can we go home now?" —MARVEA

There are times when we cannot function and we need to withdraw and regroup. There are situations that we know we cannot handle. In spite of all the pushing and urging of friends and family who insist that we will have a wonderful time, the patient senses that it will lead to his mental devastation. If I do not listen to my body and withdraw from the overstimulation, it takes several days for my intellectual abilities to return. This is very frightening because I can't help wondering each time this happens if I've pushed myself totally over the line of no return.

—Excerpt from *My Journey into Alzheimer's Disease* by Robert Davis

It may take two weeks to recover from one family reunion, and the caregiver suffers the repercussions. Spread holidays throughout the year. On Sunday, go to the Christmas church service. The next week invite one family for dinner. The next month open presents.

Rethink the holiday traditions:

* Call a family meeting before the holidays. Discuss traditions that must be continued and ones that can be changed.
* It is *not* a choice; the caregiver *needs* help. If the caregiver insists on cooking the turkey and favorite stuffing, you buy the turkey and ingredients for stuffing. Ask each guest to bring a vegetable.
* During the family get-together, be sure the person is seated in their place of comfort or next to their favorite family member who is assisting. Say: "Here comes Annie. Dinner is almost ready."
* If the person is restless, have someone who is attuned to the person's mood take them outside for a walk, or to the bedroom for a nap or some much needed quiet time.
* Make sure the person is never left alone in a crowd.
* Put something in the person's hands or lap (a plate of finger food, a loved pet, a baby) to create a positive distraction from the noise and stimulation.
* Put the caregiver and the person with dementia first. The rest of the family can adjust.
* Take turns being with the person with dementia. The other family members can get quality time with Dad/Mom and do what "normally" is done (shopping, eating out, watching a football game together).

I have been in Sane. They don't have an airport; you have to be driven there. I have made several trips there, thanks to my family. —Sister Agnes, S.P.

Newfound Traditions

People Stop Visiting

People stop visiting because…they don't know how to. For the past forty years, as a neighbor, as a daughter, as a friend, they have been visiting with, "What did you do this morning?" or "What did you have for lunch?" Can the person with short-term memory loss answer these questions? *No.* Then to test the person, the visitor will add, "Do you remember the drive I took you on yesterday?" *No,* they don't remember the drive, and the confusion increases. When the confusion increases, how do you think it makes the visitor and the person with dementia feel? Uncomfortable.

People also stop visiting because they are scared of the diagnosis. We have our own perception of what it means to have Alzheimer's and "lose your mind." In the past, it meant you were "crazy." You may have seen your neighbor walk outside naked. You may have witnessed your grandpa being "hauled off." You may have seen something on the Internet about how "they" get violent. Whatever the perception, the underlying emotion is fear. Fear of what this person will look like and how they will act. Our fear is far worse than our actual experience.

Friends and family have a tough time visiting because they can't stand seeing him this way, because he is not the way he was. They pity him because if he knew how he was, he wouldn't want to live this way. I know they would rather remember him the way he used to be. —MARVEA

One of the ways to change the perception, and one of the greatest gifts we can give, is to teach friends and family "how to visit."

Dear friends and family,

As you know, Lee has Alzheimer's and it is getting more difficult for us to visit you. We treasure your relationship so here are some tips for visiting us.

Lee has good days and difficult days. If possible, please call ahead of time. If it seems to be a difficult day, just drop off whatever you have brought. On a good day, stay and enjoy your time, but I may use this time to excuse myself to get some "me" time.

As much as you would like to come as a family, please only one or two people at a time. Three or more is too overwhelming and too much noise, which he very sensitive to. If you talk loudly, don't be surprised if he hollers back in irritation.

Greet Lee with a hug or handshake. He loves personal touch and he will like you instantly if you bring him...apple pie with vanilla ice cream, the newspaper, popcorn, a calendar of old cars, or a bag of Werther's candies.

He still loves to work, and as you know he could fix about anything. Now he isn't able to fix things, but he still enjoys tinkering on his motors and will show off his 350 engine in the garage. If he is having a good day, work on the yard together, and share a Dr. Pepper. I have plenty of Dr. Pepper.

He loves to go for car rides. Play old country music, or just enjoy the quiet. You know Lee—he never really was a talker. If you take him out to eat without me, avoid the lunch hour rush and ask me before you leave what to order for him. He cannot make choices—it just upsets him.

He likes to be a part of the conversation and still contributes. When he repeats his story, simply be polite. Lee has difficulty with words, so if you don't understand what he is saying just agree and say, "You're a Smidt," which implies he is still very smart.

Please avoid questions that require him to use his short-term memory, like, "What did you do this morning?" or starting with, "Do you remember...?" Instead, chat about what you have been doing. If he gets frustrated, just eat the apple pie. Anything sweet will shift his mood.

If you have any old pictures of Lee with family and friends, bring a copy and simply give him his memory back. A picture may prompt him to tell you a story you haven't heard before.

Thank you for adjusting to this new world we find ourselves in. Every day is a new day, and we hope we can navigate it together.

With our love and appreciation,
Joan and Lee

The Visit

A hug, a handshake, and a smile.
He looks at you and says, "I haven't seen you in a while."
He said the same thing when you saw him yesterday.
You smile at him and know, the visit will be okay.
You look at him, fighting back the tears.
He doesn't remember he has known you for years and years.
A short visit and he is as happy as can be.
He says, to no one in particular, "Who is that person?
So glad he came to visit me!"

—Marvea

Piglet sidled up to Pooh from behind. "Pooh!" he whispered. "Yes, Piglet?" "Nothing," said Piglet, taking Pooh's paw. "I just wanted to be sure of you." —A.A. MILNE

Newfound Visit

Not Forgotten

This person may not recognize you, but he or she has not forgotten you. When we say, "She won't remember you," we are giving a hopeless message. Alzheimer's is not hopeless. Understand that she may not recognize you because she thinks of you as a child, or a young handsome beau.

> Bud and his wife who has Alzheimer's went to the park where they used to "go parking" as teenagers. He leaned over, touched her cheek, and said, "I love you." She said, "I'm sorry sir, but my heart is for Bud." He can think, "She doesn't know me." Or he can smile and say, "She still loves me!!!"

They may not recognize your face, but far into the disease they will recognize your voice.

> A son went to visit his mom. While walking down the hall he called out, "Mom!" She replied, "Larry! Larry!" But as soon as the son was close enough for her to see, she didn't know who he was.

> During their visits she would stand behind her brother, rub his back, and give him childhood memories. They chatted, but when she came around to the front and he saw her face, he would be confused.

> During the day Mom sometimes swears at me because she's mad that I did this or that. But at night when I sit beside her bed and hold her hand, she will turn to me and say, "Where have you been?" I am her daughter again.

Families stop visiting because, "What's the point, the person doesn't know who I am." They may not know who you are, but you know who they are. So daughters and sons, when you visit your mom or dad, bring a picture of yourself at the age they believe you to be. Kneel down to become small. They may have a moment of recollection because they see you as a child. Instead of saying, "Dad, do you remember me?," as soon as you say "Dad," he is wondering who you are. When you say, "Do you remember…?" you are setting him up to fail. Instead, say his first name: "John, I found this picture of your son, Ryan. He loves to play baseball too." Who is the best person to give memories of Ryan back to his dad? Ryan. You never know, Ryan might hear stories about himself that he has never heard before. His dad might point at the picture and say, "I love my boy."

I have been fighting with mom for the last twenty years. I now introduce myself to my mom and say, "Hi, Margaret. I was hoping you could tell me about the little blond girl in this picture." My mom tells me stories filled with love and adoration for this little girl. These moments have replaced my anger.

A daughter explained to me how she grew up with four brothers and she was the only girl. She and her father had never been very close. After he was diagnosed with Alzheimer's, she became his caregiver. She confided to me that she is getting to know her dad for the first time because he doesn't recognize her.

Parents tell everyone else about their kid. When you become a friend or visitor, they're more likely to tell you things you never knew about yourself. You might learn something about your parents you didn't want to know. Consider the blessing of getting to know them more fully.

Ohana means family. Family means nobody gets left behind or forgotten. —LILO AND STITCH

Newfound Child

"Who Are You?"

He thinks you're his wife, but you're his daughter. She thinks you're Mom, but you're her sister. He thinks you're his daughter, but you're his granddaughter. He thinks you're a stranger, but you're his friend. Be whomever they want you to be.

Imagine a husband is trying to take care of his wife at home and in this moment she doesn't know who he is. How does that make her feel? Threatened and wondering when is he going to leave. Then the husband tries to reason with his wife: "We have been married for sixty-two years. I love you." She screams back, "Get the #%$***% out of my house, you $%**#%." If he doesn't leave she will go over to the neighbor's house and call the police.

How does this make her husband, who doesn't understand this disease, feel? Horrible. It's important to have men-specific support groups because then and only then can men open up about the trials and tribulations they are personally facing.

I have met some husbands who are pretty darn smart, and they've shared these suggestions:

When my wife doesn't know who I am, I simply let her know I am the plumber and I am there to fix her sink. She isn't threatened by a plumber.

When my wife wants me but doesn't recognize me, I simply step outside for five minutes and come through the front door with my normal greeting. "Honey, I'm home! I am headed to the garage." As long as she doesn't see my face she recognizes my voice, and therefore I am home.

I figured out that if I shut the light off before I go to bed, I can be whomever she wants me to be. (Where did she find him? We all want a man like that.)

Turn this around and imagine that the husband has Alzheimer's and his wife is taking care of him. He looks over and sees this older lady. First thought: "Church lady, good food." He is not threatened by her.

When children and their spouses visit, often the person will recognize the spouse but not their own son or daughter. Why? Because they have only known their child's spouse as an adult. How does a son feel when his mother wonders who he is but calls his spouse by name? Forgotten. But he's not forgotten. He is simply too old to be her son.

My mother truly "hits" on my husband. He loves the extra attention and plays right along.

When my dad becomes upset, I just become his secretary because he always had a secretary. I get a pad and pencil, sit down in front of him, and ask very simple questions at first. Soon his words become sentences and his sentences become paragraphs. Being his secretary gives me my dad back.

"My father-in-law moved in with us and has been making advances toward me. It's extremely awkward. What do I do?" My suggestion: "Don't be so cute. Dress frumpy. Maybe the only solution is to allow someone else to care for him. He is a man and you're a beautiful woman."

A grandpa was making advances toward his teenage granddaughter, who looked like her grandmother. We can call this "inappropriate," but he is still attracted to his girlfriend in his teenage mind.

There is a gentleman who loves to dance. I call him "Pa," and he calls me "Ma." I tell him, "It's Friday night, and we're going dancing. First we'll stop at Red's" (a bar that used to be in town). "Then we'll go dancing." It brings a smile to his face every time. The next day, I ask him if he's tired because we danced all night. He smiles from ear to ear. —LUONNE WHITFORD

A gentleman came up and gave me a big hug, telling me it had been so long since he had seen me. I replied, "Yes, it has. It's so good to see you." Then a caregiver came up and said, "Bob, this lady is just visiting. It's not..." I wanted to say, "Stop it!!!" I could've been his long-lost friend. I could've been his neighbor. I could've been his sister and we could've chatted like old times.

My mom thinks I am my dad and calls me by his name. I simply change my attire by putting on an old T-shirt and ball cap so I look more like her boy.

You see, dementia gave me the mother I have always wanted. She loves my
clothes, my hair, my face, my voice, and she lights up every time I visit.

—Sharon Snir

If someone doesn't like you, consider that you probably look like someone they never liked. Don't take it personally, because you might look like the person they believe is having an affair with their spouse.

My mom won't leave my dad because he constantly accuses her of having an
affair. My brothers can no longer visit because my dad thinks they are the
"other man." My suggestion: Dad is going to have this story whether she
is standing in front of him or she is out getting her hair done. Same result,
different benefits. So take her out to get her hair done. As for your brothers,
make sure they visit with a woman on their arm so they "look" married. Or
have them look like the TV repairman. Or have them dress up like a woman.
How far you can role-play so this person isn't threatened by you. ☺

Accusing their spouse of having an affair is very common. If they don't recognize you in this moment, then where are you? Any undercurrent of a past fear will be exacerbated in the dementia. Whether the fear is warranted or not, if it has ever spun in their head, it will now be fully expressed out loud. You may have never been unfaithful, but they will accuse you because it is their story, their fear. Maybe you were unfaithful years ago and thought it had been resolved, but it resurfaces with the same intensity, as if it were happening all over again. Let the person fully express themselves again and again. It simply needs to come out. Then apologize for your actions and ask for forgiveness.

I met a gentleman who believed that the reason marriages were failing today is
because men stop courting their wives. He continued, "I can no longer court
my wife because she doesn't know who I am." With a big smile I replied, "Oh
yes you can. Write her love letters to read over and over again. Call her on the
phone and tell her, 'It's John, and I'm the luckiest guy in the world to have a
beautiful girl like you.' And send her flowers so she's reminded of your love.
Court your wife again."

For all you men out there… court your woman again. Send love letters, flowers, and visuals so she can be assured of your love, even when you are not there.

All the world is a stage and all the men and women merely players. —WILLIAM SHAKESPEARE

Newfound You

What
Do You Love?

Reading: Read out loud to them
Singing: Sing for them
Watching birds: Bring a video of baby bluebirds
Cleaning: However they help, say "Thank you"
Playing the saxophone: Play on
Makeup: Do their makeup
Poetry: They are your audience
Nibbling: Nibble together
Baking: Roll out the dough
Your dogs: Bring in videos of them playing
Your kids: Bring them with you
Doing nothing: Wrap them up in soft blanket
and put your feet up together

Whatever you love to do, do that with someone.

What Does
This Person Love?

Traveling: Download sounds and pictures from the Internet
Fishing: Clean out tackle box 'n' fry some fish together
Mail: Copy letters received over the years
(birthday cards, love letters, postcards)
Gardening: Dig holes
Baking: Sift flour
Tea: Have a tea party
Download sounds from their childhood:
Farm kid—A rooster crowing, birds chirping, dog
barking, cows mooing, screen door slamming
with a picture of Grandma's house
City kid—Horns honking, subway racket, ice
cream truck jingle or carnival noises

If they are doing what they love, it will be easy to do.

You've Got Mail!

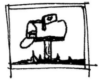

How does it feel to get a package or letter in the mail? Oh so good! If a family member or friend doesn't feel comfortable visiting or cannot visit, pop something in the mail. They will read a card over and over again, especially if you add old pictures with your memories written on the back.

> *A lady once said to me, "I have known my friend since we were children. We even lived together for ten years and have continued writing even though we are miles apart. My friend stopped writing because of Alzheimer's. Would it do any good to continue to write?" My response to her was, "Yes! You must continue to write. You are her memory." I was fortunate enough to meet this lady again and she shared with me her wonderful story. "I wrote long letters to my friend telling her of our funny moments, our adventurous moments, and our quiet moments from long ago. I also sent her pictures that we had taken together in our younger days. I did not hear back from her, but her daughters called me and said the letters brought laughter, tears, and joy. The daughters heard stories they never knew about their mom. I was filled with such joy to know I brought moments of joy to my dear friend."*

Bring cards that say, "Thinking about you," "You're a special friend," or "Hello," and sign them, "From your Loving Family." No matter who picks the card up, they will think it's for them. Send a package and enclose some pretty jewelry, candy, poems, perfume, fishing lures, Ponds Cold Cream, or other fun things.

> *My mom lives in another state and I sent her a little package of Kleenex every week (to stuff up her sleeve as she always did) and a note. The caregiver told me it makes her smile.*

Continue to put the person's address on the church mailing list so they still feel a part of their "church community." If the person lives or lived in a small town in their younger years, order their community newspaper. Do not subscribe to city newspapers, though, as bad news can be extremely confusing.

Send a magazine subscription on a subject they enjoy. It's not about the words, so be sure it's filled with beautiful pictures.

A care community can "create" mail by recycling unwanted junk mail, magazines, or newspapers. Of course, have a mailbox and ask someone to deliver the mail.

Write a letter with them and ask what they would like to say. Encourage the person to sign their name because they are able to write their signature far into the disease.

Before Mother's Day, I helped the ladies send letters to their children. A daughter, with tears in her eyes, found me and simply said, "Thank you. My mom's letter meant so much to me. I haven't received a letter from her in so long."

Go home, copy your love letters, and sprinkle them in a memory care community. If you have children, have them draw pictures. Seeing a child's drawing makes us all smile. Dig up those old postcards or Christmas cards you have saved for…what? For this very reason…to pass on…because boxes of letters and old cards are sure to create joy.

Snail mail is an unexpected party in a letter. —UNKNOWN

Newfound Message

Challenging Moments

Take things lightly and you will fly. —Jolene

Development Level

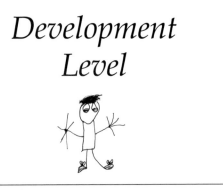

In the early stages of Alzheimer's, their developmental level is that of an eight- to ten-year-old child. As the disease progresses, their developmental level will regress to age five or younger. This is not the age they believe they are living in their mind, this is what they are able to comprehend and understand. Then in the late stages of Alzheimer's, their developmental level regresses to that of an infant.

What's one of the first words a child says? *No.* What is one of the last words a person with dementia can say? *No.* "Do you need to use the bathroom?" "No." "Do you need a nap?" "No." Stop asking the question; the answer will be "No." Turn your question around: "Let's use the bathroom before we eat." "Let's take a nap. I'm tired." Like a toddler, when they don't have words, communication is expressed with body language and outward emotions (cries, tantrums, hitting). The only way to tell you to stop or to back off is to hit. It's not a behavior, it's a reaction.

Now think about clothing and how that corresponds to a child's developmental stage. At what age does your child want to wear the same outfit every day? Four to six, when they get a new outfit for preschool. At what age does your child wear clothes inside out, only underwear, or purple with green? Around age three. At what age does your child love to be naked, come into the living room, and point their heinie at you? Three and younger. (Oh wait…all the way up to ten years old??? When does it end?)

The person with Alzheimer's will regress to wearing the same outfit seven days a week, then to wearing a bra over four blouses and clothes that don't fit and aren't theirs. Eventually they will walk completely naked into the middle of the living room, filled with people, and think nothing of it. They lose their inhibitions as a child gains their inhibitions.

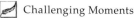

Being naked

Being naked is common, and if no one is getting hurt, let it go. If they were in a care community, know that when you put clothes on that man, the women are going to miss him. "Oh my God, did you see that man?!?" Gossiping is a healthy activity. If you must get the person dressed: have a fan blow on them, or when it's winter open the door and have a robe handy because, "Brrr…it's cold." There are jumpsuits you can get on the Internet that button up the back. You can also sew on the buttons permanently or on the inside of the seam so the person doesn't see them. (But consider it feels good to be naked. Have you tried it lately?☺)

An early-onset lady who was a speed walker was often naked. Family bought her jogging suits in her favorite color. Caregivers said, "Time to get dressed to speed walk." She would get dressed. "Speed walk" triggered her to get dressed.

Word vomit

When a child is thinking something, do they have the ability to say, "Should I say that?" No. Whatever they're thinking comes right out of their mouth. The person with dementia is the same way. Quite possibly, the person has been stuffing their emotions for a lifetime and now gets to let it all out!

Betty retorted with a solemn straight face, "Some sit there like dumb clucks, in their own importance and when they speak it's like…[then she mouthed] "Wah, wah, wah." (Consider they say what we want to say.☺)

Structure and routine

A person with dementia needs structure and routine, just as children do. When people are busy their minds are calm and more focused. When children aren't busy, what do they get into? Trouble. (Skip to the chapter "Sundowning" for more tips.)

One task at a time

When eating…eat with them. When putting on a sock…focus on the sock while touching their foot. Instead of preparing a salad…tear lettuce. Instead of clearing the table…wipe place mats. Instead of cleaning the house…sweep. Instead of three people in a conversation…let it be just you and them. Instead of music while exercising…lift your arms with them. One instruction; one thing happening at a time.

Simplify, simplify, simplify

If the person is struggling, simplify whatever you are doing to the level at which your three-year-old child would succeed.

When my daughter was three, she asked if she could help me clear the dishwasher. "No!" She might break my dishes, but she could sort the silverware. People with dementia can sort silverware too.

She began to need help dressing. Panty hose were the biggest problem. I wish I had kept notes of all the things one can do wrong when putting on panty hose. Very soon that was no longer a problem. We did away with panty hose and changed to knee-high socks. Brassieres were the next to go. There are lots of ways to simplify, and it's not all bad. —PAUL EDWARDS, HUSBAND AND CAREGIVER

Tone of voice

Your tone of voice matters. Lower your register; high pitches are irritating. Your tone of voice denotes respect or condescension. No matter whether you're speaking with a child or an older person, speak with respect.

Fewer words

They get to a place where they don't understand a word coming out of your mouth.

When my husband and I go into public and people are talking, he says, "Gobble, gobble, gobble." (Ding, ding! Consider that we people gobble a lot!)

Demonstrate

Replace your words with visuals. If they don't understand your words, demonstrate what you are wanting them to do.

A caregiver was trying to get a gentleman to take out his dentures. This had become a daily struggle. Finally, she pulled out her dentures. It worked! He then took out his.

A caregiver struggled to put Depends on a person, so she put one on herself. The person not only cooperated, but her attitude changed about wearing a Depends. (Better to call it underwear.)

Need a nap

When a child doesn't get a nap, how are they at the end of the day? Cranky, confused, and unreasonable. When a person with dementia doesn't get enough rest, how are they? Naps, naps, naps!

Everything goes in their mouth

When my son was one and playing in the sand pile, he would shovel sand into his mouth like candy. I thought of Dowell; in the late stages of his dementia, he would eat flowers and dirt. Understand his developmental level. He puts everything in his mouth, so replace the dirt with finger food.

If you put lotion in their hands, they might try to lick it off. Too often we jump to the conclusion this person cannot have lotion anymore. I disagree. It is our responsibility to kick-start the motion and rub it in.

Let go of your expectations

My mom would crawl on the floor. I continually tried to get her to walk. She would just bend down and crawl again. When I realized her developmental level was that of a one-year-old child, I changed the way I interacted with her in every aspect.

Because their developmental level is that of a child, they will act like a child. With other children they will fight over something they both want. They will be snotty to one another, or they may get along beautifully.

If you understand children, you will be a wonderful nutty caregiver. What works for children will probably work for this person. Personally, I tried things out on my kids first before I used these ideas at work.

The child [the older person], the one that irritates you the most, love them just as much as the other children. —S. Mary Ann, a teacher's advice

---

Newfound Development

Live Their Truth

Y ou were taught not to lie to your parents under normal circumstances, but these are not normal circumstances. This is a disease that has made this time (younger) in their life their truth. They cannot change their truth no matter how many times you correct them. All you have is this moment. What is the most loving thing to do in this moment? Make them feel better: "Mom will be right back." Or make them feel worse: "You're mom is no longer living." Keep changing your answer until you find the one that makes this person feel like everything is perfectly okay.

"Where is my mom?"
"Your mom's in the garden."
"Your mom's making dinner."
"Your mom's visiting her sister."
"Your mom will be right back."

You might think their mom would be at work or shopping. But in their generation mothers didn't usually go to work or go shopping. When our generation gets dementia, our moms will be working and shopping.

We tried everything, but nothing worked for this lady. Finally we asked her son where his mom's mom would be during the day. He explained that his mom grew up in a boarding school and her mom would visit on the weekend. We found a treasure: "Your mom is coming to see you this weekend."

"Where are my children?"
"Your baby is sleeping."
"Your kids are in school."
"Sue is taking a nap."
"Tom is doing his chores."

If she thinks her kids are older:

*Sarah would ask fifty times a day, "Where are my children?" Now we knew Sarah had a strong work ethic, so the answer that usually worked was, "Ted is working downtown, and Shirley will pick you up at 5:00 p.m." Ted actually did work downtown, and if Sarah had a good morning she would be okay with Shirley picking her up at 5:00. If she wasn't having a good day, she would usually respond, "I raised and took care of those kids; they better take care of me. I am not staying here until 5:00." Because of her short-term memory loss she would come around the corner within thirty seconds and ask the same question to the same person. If she was upset, we knew we needed to change our response. "Ted is at work, and Shirley just called and said she is picking you up at 10:00 this morning." Then at 10:00 we would say, "Shirley is picking you up at 12:00"; at 12:00, "She is picking you up at 4:00"; at 4:00, "She is picking you up after supper"; after supper, "She is picking you up at 8:00"; at 8:00, "She is picking you up in the morning." By now, you probably realize Shirley isn't going to pick her up. Shirley isn't picking her up until Tuesday to take her out for lunch, but that answer, to say the least, upset Sarah. Sarah was **okay** with staying a little longer, but she wasn't going to stay here until Tuesday!*

"Where is my wife?"

"Alice is at church."

"Alice is getting her hair done."

"Alice is playing bridge."

"Your wife will be here soon."

The reason many of your answers do not work is because you say: "He's uptown," "She's outside." The person with dementia doesn't know who you are talking about when you say *he, she, they* or *it*. Saying a person's first name triggers a response.

My husband has Alzheimer's. We used to routinely do dishes together after every meal. When I say, "I need your help with the dishes," my husband doesn't get up. But when I say, "Sharon needs your help with the dishes," my husband will get up and help me. —SHARON

"Where is my husband?"

"Joe is at work."

"Joe is uptown with Fred."

"Joe is out in the field."

"Joe is at the hardware store."

"Joe went to get the paper."

If you say, "Joe is at church," and she gives you a look like, "Liar," when she comes around the corner again asking for her husband you might want to change your answer. "Joe is at the bar." She might be ticked off because he is at the bar again but it is the answer she believes, so being ticked off is a normal reaction. Now become her girlfriend and let her vent about what a big jerk he is.

"I have to go to work."

"It's Saturday." (Not knowing what day it is becomes a blessing, because it can be Saturday every single day of the week. P.S., "It's Saturday" won't work for a farmer.)

"It's a holiday."

"The boss called and won't be in. He said to take the day off."

"The road is out." (Even if they fix the road going into town, the road is forever out.)

"There's a bad storm coming."

"I need to go to school."

"They canceled school."

"It's summer vacation."

"Okay, let's get dressed."

If you hesitate they won't believe the answer that comes out of your mouth. Ninety percent of what they understand is not the words you use but how you say it and your facial expression.

Keep answers short and simple. When the person is losing their ability to communicate, they can't understand if your answer goes into two or more sentences, you will lose 'em.

"Chuck did the chores."

"I just milked Bessie."

"Judy is taking care of your cat."

"Bill is checking on your home."

"All your bills are paid." (Give them a statement: "paid in full.")

"Your son John needed to borrow the car."

Every person is different, so some of these answers will work and some won't. When you find the answer that works, tell everyone! Keep a notebook with some blank pages so when someone finds something that works, they too can write it down for everyone to use.

It was time to get Dad ready for respite care, which was always a challenge. Dad was comfortable in his bed and I told him that I was getting dressed for a meeting at the church and he could go with me. Trying not to tell him what to do, I told him I was leaving in an hour. To my surprise he got up and got dressed. I noticed Dad was putting on his nicest gray suit with a perfectly starched white shirt. And he was tying his red tie like he had done for thirty years as a successful banker. Before today I would have asked him why he was wearing a suit and where he thought we were going. Today I tried a different approach. I told him they just called to say we shouldn't wear a coat and tie today and I wasn't going to wear one either. Having heard me say the word "church," he asked why we wouldn't wear a suit to a wedding. I paused and thought again. I told Dad that "the wedding" wasn't until tomorrow and we were just going to the church for a meeting. He slowly took off his coat and tie and we walked out the door. He was still the best-dressed man at respite care that day, as always. —CHUCK HUGHES, PILOT AND SON

Being loving to a person sometimes means withholding or bending the truth. Would it be more loving to correct them: "No, we're not going to a wedding." Or would it be more loving to bend the truth?

Some call this therapeutic fibbing. I still prefer to call it living in their truth because this is a disease that has made these stories their truth.

Everyone has their own version of reality. Folks with dementia have a reality that is just as valid as mine, and I treat them as I would like to be treated. —KAREN

I don't break rules, I just bend them to match what I need. —KEEGAN (MY BOY)

Newfound Truth

"I Want to Go Home"

Think about the person you know with Alzheimer's. Think about where they're sitting. Where they're sitting, does it look, feel, and smell like the home they're looking for? They only know what they see right now. When they say, "I want to go home," and we respond with, "No, you live here now. This is your home. Remember?," they want to dart out the door as soon you turn your back because they think you are *crazy*.

When they say, "I want to go home," change your response: "Please stay for some dessert." We all can stay longer for dessert. Give them the hope that they can go home, but give them a reason to stay here a little bit longer. The person can live in a place for two years and think it has been one day, one hour…That is why this works.

"I want to go home."

"How about breakfast first?"

"I want to go home."

"I just put on a pot of coffee."

"I want to go home."

"Okay, let's get dressed."

"I want to go home."

"Let me do your hair before you go."

"I want to go home."

"We are going to read devotions soon."

"I want to go home."

"The church ladies made us roast beef and mashed potatoes." (This triggers three responses: the food is good, the food is free, it would be rude if they left.)

"I want to go home."

> "We are going to sing this afternoon. I love your alto voice." (This only works if this person likes to sing. If they haven't sung a note, they are still thinking, "Crap, I gotta get out of here!")

What would be a reason they would understand to want to stay a little bit longer? Why she would want to stay is completely different than why he would want to stay. Men are much more difficult to get to stay. Women can sit and gab, but men have to be working, working, working.

When a man wants to leave, become the damsel in distress: "Would you help me with this really heavy box?" Take that man's arm, and don't be surprised when you're walking and he thinks, "Dang…Where did I find this woman?" Walking with you is a moment of joy. You might not have to get to the box because he's so distracted.

At 3:30 in the afternoon the ladies will say, "It's been lovely dear, but I really must go." The kids will be getting off the bus soon, or she needs to make supper.

Each afternoon this lady would become "agitated" and "combative." Not until a staff person sat where this lady was sitting did staff see what she was seeing: school buses stopping and kids getting off. They then understood that she was worried about her kids getting home and she wasn't there. When they closed the blinds, she was no longer agitated. (It can be that simple. Get behind their eyes—see what they are seeing.)

Figure out who she's worried about. If she's worried about her kids, ask her grown kids where they would have been after school if they weren't at home. Get the name of the friend Mom liked and trusted, or an extracurricular activity she was proud of: "Sally is playing at Ruby's house," or "Sally is at band practice." Specific names and places make all the difference in whether or not she will feel okay about staying a little longer.

If she is worried about her husband: "Bob just called and said he has to work late." Ask her husband what he did after work when he didn't come home right away. Again, get the names of his friends, because if you say, "Bob's uptown having coffee with a friend," she is questioning, "Who's the friend? Bob doesn't didn't drink coffee. You're covering for him." It's better to say, "Bob is having a beer with John."

At night when they look around the room, do they know where they are? No. Who are they worried about? Their mom not knowing where they are, their kids not knowing where they are, or their husband not knowing where they are.

"Your mom just called and she said it is too dark to walk home."

"Bob just called; the car broke down. He will pick you up in the morning."

"Sally is staying at Grandma's tonight."

I found a lady crying and asked her what was wrong. She told me she snuck out of the house, fell asleep, and was afraid her mom would be mad. I replied, "Guess what, I called your mom and told her you were staying the night with me!" She thanked me over and over. After about ten minutes, she went back to sleep...happy.　　　　　　　　　　　　　—WENDA K. GODFREY

When you say the person they are worried about "just called," that let's them know mom/husband/kids know where they are, which allows this person to relax in this moment.

When I walked into my dad's room in memory care he was all packed up, unshaven, and ready to go home as always. My trying to unpack his things always spins him out. That day I tried a different approach. I knew his razor was probably at the bottom of his packed clothes...so I told him I left "my" electric razor in his room on my last visit. I asked if I could look in the packed box for it. He said that I could. So he helped me unpack his stuff and I easily found the razor. I asked him if he had ever tried one like this. He said he hadn't. I then told him it was the best razor I had ever tried and asked him if he would like to give it a shot. He did. I asked him if I could leave it in his room so I would have one when I visited. He told me that would be fine but not to forget it tomorrow. Tomorrow I just might forget...No spin today, phew.　　　　　　　　　—CHUCK HUGHES, PILOT AND SON

Packing to "go home" is very common, especially if they have just moved into a community. Does it physically hurt anyone having all their stuff packed by the door? Nope. So let it go. This gives them the hope they can still go home.

The guilt families/spouses feel when they see the person packed and ready to "go home " sometimes compels them to move the person back home. The person may be here because the spouse had a stroke while taking care of them. Once the spouse is better they are determined to bring them home and take care of them again. Again they will end up in the hospital.

Even if families take them home, the person will still "want to go home." The home they're looking for is the home they were living in at the age at which they are living in their mind. They will walk out of a house they have lived in for forty years, thinking they're just visiting.

My husband, Bob, would tell me he had to go home. I would literally have to get him in the car, take him up the road, come back by the house, and have him tell me where the house was. Then he was fine for the rest of the night.

—Shirley Larsen

Home is also a feeling. When they feel loved and accepted, they are more likely to feel at "home." Just love 'em, just love 'em.

Find the lead from the unfamiliar to the familiar. —Sister Ellen, S.P.

Newfound Home

Stop Correcting Them

First, let's give you Alzheimer's so you know how it feels. Poof! You have Alzheimer's, and you're in a room that you don't recognize (but you actually live there). You see your purse and pick it up. Someone comes along, takes it, and says, "That's not your purse, Alice."

Then you walk into a room, and lying on the chair is your sweater. You put it on and it feels so good to be warm. As you are walking out of the room, someone comes up to you and says, "Alice, that is Edith's sweater." They take your sweater.

You're a bit tired and you see this nice comfy chair in another room. You sit down, and suddenly someone yells, "Get out of my room! Get out of my room!" And you get caned on the way out.

Now you just want to go home, so you walk toward the door. Someone says, "Alice, don't go down there." You push on the door and an alarm sounds. You walk to another door. It's locked. You ask the next person you see, "Will you take me home? I live at 1200 Phillips Street." They tell you, "You live here now." You start to panic: "I gotta get out of here!"

This is how they feel. They don't know they're doing anything wrong until we show up and correct them. They aren't even confused until we show up!

STOP CORRECTING THEM! Would they be taking someone's stuff if they knew it wasn't theirs? *No.* Would they be wearing someone else's sweater if they knew it wasn't theirs? *No.* Would they be in someone else's room if they knew it wasn't theirs? *No.* No matter how many times we correct them, can they change? *No.* Again, guess who has to be the one to change? Yes, it's still you.

A lady approached me after a presentation and said, "Because of you, I am going to let my mom wear her nightgown every day and with no underwear underneath it." I said, "I hope so." Continuing on, she said, "Because what you are saying is that I am tired of fighting with her." I said, "I hope so."

Before you correct someone, pause and ask yourself three questions. Let's just use one of the toughest examples: wearing the same outfit every single day.

First question: Does it hurt you physically (not annoy you—we are easily annoyed) that they wear the same outfit every day? If you are answering honestly, the answer is "No."

Second question: Does it physically hurt any of the other people living here? "No." (When you get older you lose your sense of smell.)

Third question: Does it hurt the person with dementia physically to wear the same outfit every single day? "No."

If you answered "No" to these three questions, let it go. It's difficult enough to get dressed once a day, let alone twice.

Even if the outfit is dirty or has an odor, does it physically hurt anyone? *No.* If the outfit is soiled, then yes, now is the time to give them a reason to change clothes: "Company is coming." "It's Saturday night." "Let's get cleaned up for church." Simply give them a reason they would understand to get "washed up."

Since they have short-term memory loss, do they remember wearing that outfit yesterday? No. Why do they choose that outfit? They like it. It makes them feel good. Allowing this choice means respecting their dignity. Don't you get to choose what outfit you wear?

Go ahead and try to throw away their favorite outfit. Do they forget about it? Absolutely not! They're mad now because they can't find it. Who suffers the repercussions? You do.

You might buy the person a whole new wardrobe in the hopes that they will wear something else: "Look at all the new clothes I bought you!" Now the person is mad because you spent their money. My suggestion: Sneak nine similar outfits into the closet and put one in a brown paper bag, saying, "I got it for ten cents at a garage sale." If the person grew up with money, put the outfit in a bag from their favorite clothing store and say, "I found it on sale and just couldn't pass it up!" In their generation, if it was inexpensive, they would wear it. If it was expensive, they would save it for a special occasion.

> *A lady only wanted to wear her blue sweatshirt with a kitty on it. The son did not like her wearing the same shirt every day, so I went to Goodwill and bought six blue sweatshirts with kittens on them. The son was happy and the lady thought she was wearing her kitten shirt every day.*
>
> —Wenda K. Godfrey

> *He has all these beautiful jackets but will only wear one. If it doesn't say medium, he won't put it on. We have bought him new slippers, exactly like his old ones, but he won't wear them because he has to save those.* —Marvea

Even if you buy ten, they most likely will continue to wear the "old one." Just know that tomorrow you will have created a moment of joy for five other people because they are wearing your mom's sweater or your dad's slippers. When they wear someone else's clothing, they think it's theirs. Never fight with them. It's a losing battle.

It is easy for me not to fight with them, but you want to correct the person in the hopes that they will get better. This is a rightful wish, but it's an illusion. This is a disease that progresses. Consider you want them to "look good" so you feel better. But, no matter how many times you correct them, do they get better? Do they change? No.

I hope that when you get irritated by what they are doing, you just think to yourself, "There he goes again." And if you correct them, you just laugh at yourself and think, "There I go again."

You cannot control the disease. You can only control your reaction to it. —Liz Ayres

---

Newfound Old Outfit

You Are Wrong...
They Are Right...

From this point on, you are wrong and the person with dementia is right. This is going to take therapy for some of you. Think about it: If you think you're right and the person you're caring for thinks they're right, what is going to happen? Conflict. Where does the stress level go? *Up.* Where does the kindness level go? *Down.* What is more important: people's happiness or being right?

Does anyone else have parents like this? My dad will say, "On Wednesday, we went to the sale barn." Mom stops him, "No, Dear, it wasn't Wednesday. It was Tuesday." Dad continues on, "We went over to Stella's and had cinnamon rolls." Mom then says, "No, Dear, it wasn't cinnamon rolls. It was coffee cake." STOP!!! Do you think my dad is going to say, "Hey, thanks. You're so smart." What is my dad feeling? *Frustrated, angry, and belittled.* Is my dad's story hurting anyone? *No.*

My mom has heard my presentation twenty times. Do you think she has changed? No. My mom's amazing, has a bachelor's degree, is super caring, and raised six kids beautifully. (Look at me, for example. ☺) I have had a one-on-one conversation with my mom about not correcting Dad, "Does it matter what day it happened on? Let's just not fight with him." Do you think she has changed? *No.* Because how many years has she been correcting my dad? Fifty-seven years. Just because I say, "Hey, let's not correct him," she can't just say, "Okay, I'll stop."

My mom has taught me a valuable lesson because I get intensely frustrated when families correct the person over and over. But when my mom can't do what I'm asking families to do, I realize that I'm going to have to be gentle with every family member I meet. It's easy for me to be with this person because I don't have expectations of who they should be. But you, as family, have expectations; you want to correct them in the hope that they will get better. Do they get better when you correct them? No.

My dad's story is pretty mild compared to some stories you will hear. Their stories will get big. *Real big!* Is their story hurting anyone? No. Simply listen. Please take the words *no, don't,* and *remember* out of your vocabulary and I guarantee you will have a better day.

"No, Mom, you live here now, and Dad has passed away."
>*Replace with:* "Dad's at the hardware store again."

"Helen, I am your husband. Don't you remember me?"
>*Replace with:* "Yeah, your husband can be pretty stubborn, but he loves you."

"No, Dad, I am your daughter."
>*Replace with:* "Julie loves to play the violin, just like you."

"Shirley, your parents are no longer living."
>*Replace with:* "Your parents love you. They wouldn't forget you."

"Mary, those aren't your clothes."
>*Replace with:* "Mary, company is coming. Let's get dressed up." Or let her wear those clothes.

"Don't you remember?"
>*Replace with:* "You're right. I forgot."

"You already told me that story."
>*Replace with:* "I love your stories!"

Now, men, doctors, and preachers still get to be right with women who have dementia, because in their generation men *thought* they were right. Men, savor the moment, because when my generation gets there, it isn't gonna be that way. 🙂

So who has a difficult time letting her dad be right? Me. We all have been playing roles for a lifetime. Be gentle as you unlearn them. Who is the one who taught me how to create moments of joy? My dad. My dad knows how to make anyone smile.

When I smile, you smile. When you smile, I smile. —JOLENE

Newfound Peace

Blame It on Something Else

Blame anything "bad" that happens on something or someone else: the boss, the nurse, the doctor, the government, the disliked neighbor, the kid that lives far, far away, etc. Or blame it on the insurance: "Insurance says that you have to…take this med, go to this appointment, have this person come help us in the morning." "You can't drive the car right now because we don't have insurance."

Incontinence

It can be very embarrassing for them to wake up in the morning and find that the bed is wet. Blame it on something else: "That roof is leaking again!" Or "That damn dog!" Now they think they didn't wet the bed, or they think, "You're stupid." Either answer they like because in their generation, when they wet the bed, they got in trouble. If the person is incontinent during the day, whisper, "You must have sat in a little water. Let's change so you feel better."

Forgetting appointments

You call ten times in the morning to remind them of a doctor's appointment and leave a written note on the refrigerator. When you arrive to pick them up, you begin by asking, "Are you ready to go to the doctor?" The person's answer: "You didn't tell me. I'm not ready to go anywhere!" Then, being only human, you lose your patience altogether and say, "I told you ten times!!!" When this happens you are only making them upset and reluctant to go with you. A much better response is to blame yourself for this misunderstanding: "Oh no, I forgot to tell you! I'm sorry. We can stop for ice cream." Focus on the "thing" they would like to do.

Would you like another little hint? Don't take the time to remind them, just apologize for "forgetting" and arrive early knowing they may need help getting ready.

If they catch you in a lie try the following:

"I'm sorry."

"I didn't mean to upset you. It won't happen again."

"I forgot. I'm sorry."

"You're right, I goofed."

"I'm sorry. I misunderstood."

"I'm sorry. Will you forgive me?"

You're the person who is caring for them; you want them to like you, to trust you, and to think you're on their side. If they think, "You did it!," repeat after me: "I'm sorry." Because it's hard to fight with someone who is sorry.

The man who smiles when things go wrong has thought of someone to blame it on. —ROBERT BLOCH

Newfound Scapegoat

Your Mood Affects Their Mood

You'd better believe it! Your mood absolutely affects their mood! If you're rushed, they're rushed. If you're upset, they're upset. If you're happy, they're more likely to be happy. What is your mood? Because, basically, you decide what kind of day you're going to get.

When I knew nothing about Alzheimer's, I would be all bubbly and hyper, talking loudly and fast. I felt like the faster I moved, the more I would get done. It didn't work. People were bouncing off the walls. Luckily, I couldn't keep up that pace, and in my tiredness I said, "I need to take a break. Relax, I'll be back in twenty minutes." I was ready to quit my job; I was exhausted. But when I returned almost everyone was still relaxed. Amazing! When my mood calmed down and I slowed down, so did they. —JOLENE

Families think they are interviewing me, but I am actually interviewing them through the person with Alzheimer's. I will not care for someone who is mean and nasty because that tells me the family is most likely mean and nasty. I can care for the person with Alzheimer's when they are difficult but not the family. My lady was upset all the time because her family always wanted something from her. —SISTER RICHARD

Check your body language. Check your facial expressions. Check your mood. What are they saying? You're human, and there are days you will be crabby. Before you enter the room think of something you *love*: flowers, a grandchild, a pet, a friend. Now embody that feeling.

A good mood is like a balloon…one little prick is all it takes to ruin it! —MINIONS

Newfound Mood

Illusion of Choice

If you open the closet door and ask, "What would you like to wear today?," they can't decide because there are too many choices. Instead, pull out two outfits: "Which one would you like to wear—the blue one or the red one?" They still may not be able to make the decision, so give them a reason to choose one of the outfits: "I like the blue dress. It brings out your beautiful blue eyes." Another way to give them the choice is to say, "How about I choose today, and you choose tomorrow?" When you are offering them something: "Would you like a piece of pie?," instead of putting it in front of them without choice, although no one is likely to refuse pie. Ask, "Would you like to sit by the window?," instead of telling them, "Sit here." If you're rearranging a room, ask their opinion: "Barb, does the rug look better over here?"

Say their name before you ask a question to help them focus: "Jim, do I part your hair on this side?" "Jean, would you like to wear these shoes?"

> When staff told Ray it was time to eat, he would usually refuse. But if they left the plate of food on the table next to him and walked away, the food would be gone when they came back.

> Frank didn't usually want to go to bed at night. So, staff guided him by saying, "I wonder where your room is? Frank, can you help me find it? Is this your door? No? Is it this door? Hey, we found it." For some reason, once he was in his room, he was easy to get into bed. The hard part was getting him there.

No one likes to be bossed around, no matter what their age.

Never laugh at your wife's choices. You are one of them. —Minions

---

Newfound Choice

My mom never swore…

My mom never wore the same outfit two days in a row…

My mom never wore fingernail polish…

My mom never would have slept with another man…

Oh honey, before she was your mama, she probably did all of those things! And even if she didn't say it out loud, she probably thought it! I believe that with this disease the person loses all pretense of who they should be and they reflect how they really feel. The shame and embarrassment families feel because of what their loved one is saying and doing is unnecessary. Swearing is a common occurrence. Get over it! Telling crazy stories that aren't true is a common occurrence. Get over it! Hiding dirty underwear in strange places is a common occurrence. Get over it! Your mom wanting to be held by a man that's not your dad. Get over it! Excuse me if I sound a bit callous, but those of us who have been caring for people with dementia for years are used to all of these "crazy things" they do. We simply see the person as funny, as ornery, or as sweet. We relish their wit and humor because they say what we want to say. You are just not used to your mom saying it.

People with Alzheimer's function at a higher level around nutty caregivers because these caregivers allow the person to simply be as they are. Consider that nutty caregivers know these people better than their own kids do. The person may prefer the nutty caregiver over their own kids. There can be jealousy or hurt when this happens. Get over it! Be glad they have someone they like and trust!

> There was a lady who wouldn't get out of bed in the morning. A nutty caregiver knew she raised chickens, so she walked into her room and crowed: "Cock-a-doodle-dooooooo!!!" The lady got up.

This is the only job where we *all* get to be *off* all day. Nutty caregivers who have a bit of dementia are really good at what they do. The ones who can start to watch a movie thinking they haven't seen it, then halfway through it starts to look familiar, yet, they want to finish it because they forgot how it ended.

When someone is wearing the same outfit seven days in a row, it's not the nutty caregiver who has a problem—it's the family members who are embarrassed because they want Mom to look good.

Here is the conversation I encourage caregivers to have with families when they don't like what's happening:

"When your Mom wears that dress, she likes it and is a bit sassy. We like that too. But…when we change her dress, she gets incredibly angry. I don't know about you, but I don't want her angry."

Do they want their mom angry? *No.* Did this conversation focus on what the family wants? *No.* Did this conversation focus on what the caregiver wants? *No.* Who does this entire conversation focus on? *The emotions of the person we all care about.*

Every conversation needs to focus on the person. Now, there's still going to be a family member who says, "I don't care. My mom never would've worn the same outfit two days in a row! Change it. This is what I am paying you to do." In that case simply respond, "Okay…let's go change her outfit together." Not until this family member experiences firsthand what the caregivers have been experiencing will they believe it's actually happening. Families will just think caregivers are being lazy. *Show families the emotions you're experiencing with this person.*

May we all get over it! Let's all allow everyone we meet to be as they are.

"Only hot flash I get is when the Ol' Man jumps in bed with me." —CONNIE, MOM

Newfound Mom

Swearing

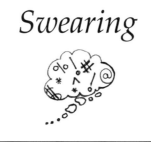

Swearing like a sailor is common, even for the sweetest of ladies. Being ashamed is unnecessary. When the person is thinking something, it will come right out their mouth. Expect them to drop the f-bomb and tell you, "You have a fat ass." If they are pissed at someone...shut the damn door and swear with them about "that bitch walking around."

A caregiving nun on an outing: "Don't say it out loud. Just keep it in. On the way home you can swear all you like." Then on the way home she let it rip: "God damn it!"

I walked up to a lady and said, "Well, don't we look sassy today." She flared back, "Oh, go to hell." I jested, "Only if you go with me!" A questionable smirk appeared on her face.

When you reprimand them by saying, "You shouldn't talk like that," do they like you? *No.* Allow the person to express themselves. If you're able, agree with their judgment: "I know! I can't believe she did that!" If they feel like you're on their side, they will like you instantly.

It's good to have a child with you because they're less likely to swear. Or just put your hair in pigtails and become the child. Make it light and say, "I can't believe you just sad that!," with a smile.

A caregiver asked me why a person she cares for might call her a bossy bitch. I asked her, "How do you approach her?" She responded, "When I come in the room I let her know she needs to get dressed. Then it's time to go to breakfast because she needs to eat." My gentle retort: "You might want to consider ..."

They are truth tellers and might see something you can't. This is the part I actually delight in because they can say the perfectly perfect one liner when you least expect it.

The lady told me to go fix my hair and when I turned to walk away she added, "Oh my God, it looks as bad from the back as it does in the front."

I was drawing a picture with a lady and I asked her if she liked my art. She replied, "Almost as good as a first grader."

Every time my fiancé and I visit my mom, she asks "Who is he?" I tell her we are getting married. Her response is, "Not if I marry him first."

—ANISSA CHASE (AKA NURSE RATCHED)

My husband walked up to a big, tall lady and said, "Oh, you're bigger than me." He also walks up to men with "big bellies" and says, "Looks like you're eating good." Oddly, when he sees a child he likes to bend over and poke them gently to tease them, and before Alzheimer's he never liked little kids.

Two handsome men walked through the door. I asked Helen to come sit down. She said, "No way. Not when I can chase these two hunks around."

Women are more likely to fight over the man in the room than swear in front of him. WE NEED MORE MALE CAREGIVERS! A lady's mood changes instantly when a man walks through the door. I think if retired men just came in and sat down, everyone's day would be easier (especially if they were in uniform 😊).

When you're in public and they say something that makes you want to crawl under a table, hand the innocent bystander a business card that states: "My mom has Alzheimer's. Please forgive her." And forgive her.

Swearing: Because sometimes "gosh darn" and "meanie head" just don't cover it. —UNKNOWN

Newfound Shit

Why did you leave me here you &%!!**!

You're spending all of my money!

Where do you think you are going you &*!!%

You took it. I know you did!

Who's that you're talking to on the phone? You're talking about me, aren't you!

The one giving the care is the one who takes all the punches. A complete stranger can walk through the door and the person will be nice and act perfectly fine for a short period of time.

I would like to address this in a less threatening fashion to help you get a better grasp on why this happens. I have a teenager at home. I hear about her from the other parents and the teachers in our community. I hear about how delightful she is, how polite she is, and how helpful she is. When I hear this I wonder, *"Who are they talking about?,"* because when she comes home, she yells at me: "I hate you! You're ruining my life!" "Don't talk to me!"

Because I've had a little therapy I am able to understand that the reason she yells at me, and only me, is because she feels *safe* expressing all her feelings to me. (Now isn't that sweet?) I also understand that her frontal lobe isn't quite developed yet, so whatever she is thinking comes right out of her mouth. My therapist encouraged me to never fight with her because you cannot reason with someone who cannot reason. Well, people with Alzheimer's have a damaged frontal lobe, so we're dealing with similar situations.

You and I may understand this, but it still hurts. It hurts to watch them smile and be nice to everyone else, only to be yelled at behind closed doors. Let me share some advice from a wife I met along the way.

My husband would verbally vomit on me every time I would visit. "Why did you leave me here, you $%**!?! Take me home!" So I went out, bought a cast, and put it on my arm. As long as I looked "well" he thought I should take him home. But when he saw that I was hurt, he was nicer to me.

People with dementia only know what they *see* right now. As long as you *look* physically well and they feel safe with you, they will vomit all over you and blame you for everything they think is happening. But when they see that you're not well, they will be more sympathetic and ask, "What happened to you?"

I say, get a neck brace, leg brace, or crutches—whatever it takes for them to see that you can't take care of them right now. Then they will have a reason to take better care of you.

> *I took my husband, who has dementia, to the movie* Frozen. *My husband loved going to the movies for the popcorn and pop. The song "Let It Go" spoke to me about my attitude toward my husband's dementia. When I would make a statement or ask a question, I didn't always get a positive response from my husband. I knew it didn't do any good to argue or disagree, so I started saying to myself "let it go."* —ROBIN MOON

> *A lady put an ad in the classifieds: "Husband Wanted." The next day she received a pile of letters, all saying the same thing: "You can have mine."*

As caregivers, we think, "I have to stay strong; I'm the only one who can do this." *Not true.* Others are very capable of taking care of this person. In fact, this person might be nicer under someone else's care. I suggest that you also show your tears; *show others you are physically and emotionally hurting.* As long as you act like you're fine you are not giving others, including the person you are taking care of, the opportunity to take care of you.

I don't insult people, I just describe them. —MINIONS

Newfound Cast

The Facts Are All Off

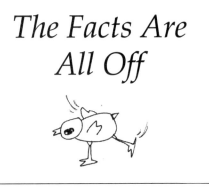

"Someone stole my mattress!"

"They are dealing drugs here!" (Which you are)

"There are whores walking around here!" (Red fingernail polish)

"There are dead people in the basement!"(TV)

"I got robbed last night!"

The facts are all off, but what they feel is right on. Respond to their feeling. If they are angry, put your hands on your hips and say to them, "That shouldn't happen! I'm going to talk to the boss!" Then leave the room in a huff. Don't go talk to the boss, just go get a drink of water. If they are scared, please don't ask what happened. That requires them to remember and talk in a complete sentence—both of which they cannot do. Simply become the protector: "I'm sorry that happened. I will check on it." Walk out the room and get a drink of water. If they say, "I got robbed last night!," respond with, "I'm calling the cops!" Don't go call the cops, just leave the room and get a drink of water. You will be highly hydrated by the end of the day.

My mom accuses me of stealing her mattress. I remind her over and over, "Why would I want your mattress?," or "I didn't take it, Mom." Not until I went out and got a mattress and leaned it up against the wall in the living room, where she could see it, did she believe that I had returned it.

If you reason with them and pat their knee saying, "I am sure no one took your stuff, but I will go look for it," they are thinking, "You did it!" By the way, they have a *rightful feeling* of being robbed because someone took their glasses, someone took their clothes to get them washed, something is missing because they hid it, and someone came in and checked on them in the middle of the night.

If they are sad, please do not ask them what's wrong. It will only make it worse. Simply bend down, put your hand on their knee, and say, "I am so sorry that happened. It shouldn't have happened." How do you know whether to hug them or not? Put your arms out wide and if they open theirs, hug them. If the person puts their head down and crosses their arms, just say, "Let it all out. I'm so sorry. Let it all out."

Angela would cry and cry and cry. We would ask, "What's wrong?," which only made her cry more. Her son eventually told us that she had been molested as a child. We changed the way we responded and let her cry, saying, "I am so sorry that happened. I am not going to let anyone hurt you."

They may also say, "My family never comes to see me. They don't love me." And you try to reason, "They were just here this weekend." Now they are fighting with you because, "No they weren't. I haven't seen my family in months!!!" Instead, respond, "I am going to call them and tell them to stop by." Don't call the family, but instead…yes, get another drink of water.

What they are feeling is real to them. Please do not try to figure out their story—respond to their feelings.

Respect people's feelings. Even though it doesn't mean anything to you, it could mean everything to them. —UNKNOWN

Newfound Feeling

"See" Authority

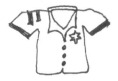

All they know is what they see right now, so I highly recommend that you have a closet with a police uniform, a doctor's jacket, a business suit, or a priest's collar (we all need forgiveness).

When they get robbed, a man in police uniform can report it. When there are spiders in their room, a man in uniform can exterminate. When they are worried about their car, a man's voice over the phone can reassure them, "The part will be in tomorrow." Every day the part will be in *tomorrow.*

When they're worried that they don't have enough money, have a man in a business suit give them a bank statement with $20,000 more than they think they have. If they don't think they can afford rent, give them a receipt and stamp in large red letters, "PAID IN FULL."

If you're a woman trying to convince them, "You have enough money—everything has already been paid for," the person will not believe you because in their generation only a man had the authority. Proof to them is a piece of paper they can hold in their hands.

If the person is verbally, physically, or emotionally hurting anyone in any way, then have a man draw the line.

A female administrator of a care community pulled me aside with tears in her eyes and shared how a male resident was verbally aggressive toward her, calling her an "f'ing bitch" whenever she walked by. I asked her if she knew a really big man. She said yes—her husband. I told her to have him put a police uniform on and confront this person by saying, "If I ever hear you talk to this woman that way again I will haul you off." Or, simply have him play the big husband protecting his wife. If this resident were in public he would not be able to talk this way.

Uniforms give the illusion of authority, and any man, whether he is retired or your neighbor down the street, can put on the uniform and handle the situation. When someone is getting hurt, no matter who they are (a wife, a child, or a resident, male or female), step in and intervene. It may even be two men fighting in a care community. Call the maintenance man. Someone has to be the man, because we as women have no authority.

A former judge was being sexually aggressive toward his female caregiver. His son would not believe his dad would talk or act that way. The caregiver asked the son to stand outside his dad's door, and not until he heard his dad making inappropriate sexual advances did he believe it was happening. I suggested to the son that he hire a male caregiver, or a not-so-pretty caregiver, and have her pull her hair back in a tight bun and wear a nurse's uniform. Not until the judge sees either a male or a woman with medical authority will he act differently.

Man's role is to be responsible and protect, first and foremost Woman, and then all of the Earth. —DUSTIN

Newfound Uniform

Everything Gets Lost

E verything, absolutely everything, gets lost—especially in the early stages, when this person thinks someone is taking their things. This only provokes them to hide more things. With short-term memory loss they don't remember where they hid things, and when they are looking for something they think, "You took it!," because they can't find it.

Go ahead, spend hours trying to find one thing; that may take weeks or months. When something comes up missing, pretend to look for it by leaving the room and let the person search for it. Is the person getting hurt while searching? *No. It's exercise.*

However, it causes great pain when diamond rings, car keys, or house keys are missing. Get ten sets of keys that work and keep them in a safe place. Get another ten sets that don't work; it's exercise for the person to try to get them to work. If the person has lost weight, their ring will easily fall off their finger. Replace the diamond with a cubic zirconia. I've seen people remove expensive items such as rings and hearing aids and wrap them in a napkin, then they get tossed in the trash. It's no one's fault. Expect it to happen. (See the chapter "Glasses Dentures Hearing Aids.")

As for purses, wallets, and canes, there is a device you can purchase on the Internet that, when something is missing, you press a button and it beeps until you locate it. You *all* want this device.

Make no mistake: She needs her purse—it's a body part. Go ahead, put it in a closet for safe keeping. Within moments she will ask where her purse is. You can reassure her over and over and over again, but she will not settle until she is actually holding her purse. As long as the purse is filled with sugar packets, apples, napkins, and silverware, she has a sense of security.

If the person is in a memory care community, *label everything* so there is the hope of it being returned, but please do not expect staff to go looking for items. Countless families have asked, "Where's the sweater I bought my mom yesterday?" STOP! Is it more important to be with people or to look for stuff? **Be with people!** Too much energy is wasted looking for stuff. Get ten sweaters; get ten purses. Know that tomorrow five will be missing, but you created a moment of joy for the five other ladies who have them.

A daughter shared with me how her dad liked baseball caps, so she ordered forty-four of his favorite team's cap. When he passed away, she only found two. We looked at each other and said, "Forty-two other people are having a moment of joy with your dad's baseball caps."

If families are asking you to look for a sweater during meal time, simply get a marker board and write it down. Let the families know that now everyone will be on the lookout, and when an item is found it will be returned (only to be lost again). Remember: Items are not "stolen," they are simply misplaced.

Unfortunately, when something gets lost families take *it* home to keep *it* safe, or the activity person puts *it* in a closet until two o'clock on Wednesday for an activity. Is *it* bringing anyone joy locked in a closet?

We have so much stuff, and the stuff they need has been thrown away, or sold at a garage sale for twenty-five cents. Families, please keep some stuff to back up the stuff that will get lost. And consider whatever you bring a donation.

Smart memory care communities have a chest of drawers in the living room filled with stuff so when anyone is missing something, the caregiver says, "I think I put it in here." Then the person gets to rummage through the drawers and take anything they like.

Brilliant idea: Go into your closet or garage and pull out stuff you no longer want, then bring joy by giving it to someone else.

There is so much we can let go of, without losing a thing. —RALPH MARSTON

Newfound Lost

Replace, Replace, Replace

S ometimes we really do need what they have. If you absolutely must take something away, replace it with something else.

When my little boy was two years old, he would get ahold of a fork or another item I didn't want him to have. I would ask him to give it to me. Well, he wouldn't. Then I would try to take it out of his hands. Did you know this little man was stronger than I? So what I would do was get out his favorite tractor and start playing with it in front of him. He would then drop the fork. We both won.

Mary was in tears and I asked her why. She pointed at my wedding ring, then in jumbled words she expressed how her husband would be upset when he found out she had lost hers. Her husband was no longer living, and her family took her ring because they didn't want her to lose it, but she could not remember that. Replace her ring.

If someone sees another person wearing her sweater and says, "That's my sweater!," don't just take the sweater away. Replace it. "Joan, this sweater would look gorgeous on you. Let's try it on!" A bit of advice: Don't ask them, "Would you like to wear this sweater?" The answer will be "No." Show the family the sweater their mom loves (pink; buttons down the front; big pockets). If you simply make a request for more sweaters, the family will buy a $100 sweater…wrong color, pullover, and needs to be dry cleaned. Families want to help—they just don't know how. It isn't about what makes *us* feel good; it is about what makes *this person* feel good.

When the person had an item that I needed, it worked much better to make them feel like the "hero" by saying, "Oh, thank you so much. You found it!" Then I would give them a hug out of thankfulness. —Bonita Dehln

After your presentation, I went home and got my grandma's pearls that she gave me and took them to her. When I placed them around her neck, my grandma teared up. Those pearls were not bringing joy to her in my jewelry box.

—A GRANDDAUGHTER'S LOVE

Again, ask yourself if what they are carrying around is hurting anyone. If your answer is no, then let them have it. If your answer is yes, then replace whatever it is you are taking away. If you take away what is in their hands and leave them with nothing…what does that feel like? Empty, lost.

Next chance you get, put something in their hands.

Don't chase them, replace them. —UNKNOWN

Newfound Replacement

Glasses Dentures Hearing Aids

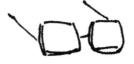

D umpster diving is a frequent event in the world of dementia. People will take out their hearing aids and dentures, or wrap their diamond ring in a napkin, and caregivers unknowingly throw them in the trash. When the person continues to take out these things, they are telling us that they don't know what they are, or that this aid is uncomfortable. The stress of losing or replacing them far outweighs the benefit. These things are only a benefit if the person knows how to use them.

We insist on taking them to the dentist or eye doctor to "fix their losses." In the early stages, yes, this makes sense, but as the disease progresses, it's literally a losing battle. Since the person can't communicate, we decide for them what we think is best. *But there is no best.* The real question is, how are they doing right now? If they seem okay, let them be as they are. Any procedure or visit to an unfamiliar place drops them into intense confusion. Is it worth it?

> *One of our residents was doing just fine with what little teeth she had left. The nursing staff persuaded the person with power of attorney that she needed dentures, and now she has had nothing but trouble when eating. Patient rights???*

> *A son was insistent that his dad get dentures, even though he was eating just fine with a few teeth. The difficult procedure and stress exacerbated the dad's dementia to the point of no return.*

On the flip side, if someone keeps their glasses on, one of the greatest gifts we can give them is to clean their glasses. Something so simple as cleaning their glasses will instantly help them function better.

When someone has a hearing loss, we think by raising our voice they may hear us. They still can't hear us, but they can see the strain on our face and become frightened by our close proximity. Do not yell to get them to hear—show them what you want to communicate. Instead of, "Do you want something to eat?," get a plate of food and see if they eat.

Focus on the senses they still have left.

Can't see, but can...
   * Feel the touch of your hand
   * Hear music with headphones
   * Hear the voice of a loved one or their dog barking
   * Taste the warmth of tea
   * Taste toast dipped in warm milk
   * Feel cozy all wrapped up

Can't hear, but can...
   * See your smile
   * See a child
   * See you twirl in your dress
   * Taste bubblegum
   * Taste warm soup from a mug
   * Feel a baby kitten
   * Feel safe with you

How can you enliven the senses they have left?

_____

I like nonsense, it wakes up the brain cells. —Dr. Seuss

Newfound Sense

Repeat, Repeat, Repeat

S hort-term memory loss allows the person to know only what they see right now. They will repeat the same question, the same story, and the same statement possibly every thirty seconds. Here are some suggestions to help you cope:

Patience, patience, patience: Patience is a virtue, but you're human and will have rough days. Guess what? Every moment is a new beginning.

Distract rather than react: Keep them busy sorting silverware and socks, folding clothes, peeling potatoes, organizing a tackle box, peeling oranges, shelling peanuts, or eating ice cream. When you find the distraction that works, then it's your turn to repeat.

Short, simple responses: "Uh huh." "Okay!" "Really?"

Listen: Without judgment. Affirm their conversation whether you agree or even understand what they are saying.

Try not to respond with, "You already told me ten times." When that slips out of your mouth then it's time for a walk, chocolate, or a chat with a friend.

My mother always says, "I don't know what I'm doing." I want to tell her, but she will forget and repeat the phrase. She loves to crochet but doesn't know what she's crocheting. The last project was about twenty-three feet long by three feet wide. She also loves to read and can't remember what she has read. It saves us money on books because she just keeps reading the same book. She loves to paint her fingernails, and that is something she can do over and over.

Repeat, repeat, repeat what they like doing. It's difficult to organize a present drawer, but they can refold wrapping paper. You unfold. She refolds.

Realize that when they verbally repeat, it's probably a statement that rolled around in their head a hundred times a day pre-dementia and now it's simply coming out their mouth. In most cases, you don't have to do anything with this thought.

A gentleman called me and shared how his wife repeated, "I don't want to live anymore. I don't want to live anymore." He had taken her to neurologists, changed her medications, and done everything in his power to give her some relief. Then at the end of our conversation he asked if he could share something with me. "Of course," I said, and then he told me this: "My wife had been having an affair for years and she knows that I know. The only thing in the past that would calm her was her martinis, but she can no longer have them because of the medication." I gently had him consider that for years she has been saying in her head, "I don't want to live anymore." Now it is simply being expressed out loud, and in this instance, martinis will give her far more relief than medication.

It's not a conclusion, it's thinking out loud. —Sister Adele Beacham, S.P.

Newfound Patience

Nonsense!

In this book I make it sound like the person with Alzheimer's is always speaking clearly, but in reality they are not. I am simply interpreting what I believe they are communicating. Often they will string together random words or phrases (making word salad), or they will replace words with other words, or they cannot find their words. When this happens you have the opportunity to consider the nonsense a delight! Few people allow themselves to experience the treat of speaking non-sensically because they are all tied up with getting to the point. But just babbling with another person can create a playful bond between you.

When two people dance, do they do it for health reasons? No! They do it because it is **fun,** and because on some level it creates a bond between them. The same can be said for having a nonsensical conversation with another person.

> *I sat down next to a lady I didn't know, and she just started babbling. I simply responded, "I know!," and laughed. Then she laughed; then I laughed some more. Then monkeys were teetering on puffy clouds with cinnamon and snowflakes. I remember resting my head on her shoulder and thanking her for this simple retreat.* —JOLENE

So the next time you feel frustrated because you don't understand a word coming out of their mouth, think **nonsense!** Think, "I get a moment when words don't matter." It's a whimsical, fly-by-the-seat-of-your-pants dance.

Monkey believes, knows, and speaks, letting the pieces, poop, and seedlings fall where they may. —PETER

Newfound Nonsense

The "Spin"

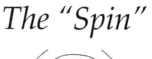

When a person is fixated on a subject that is causing much frustration, I call it a "spin" or a "loop." Believe me—you don't want to go into their spin. Simply reassure them: "That shouldn't have happened." "I'll take care of it for you." "I'll check on it." "We'll look into it."

If the person is calling 911, I can tell you they don't feel that you are taking care of it. You might think it's important to get to the bottom of the person's spin so you can help resolve their problem, but the spin will only get bigger and bigger and bigger. To get people out of the spin:

* Double over and say, "My stomach hurts!" Their mother mode will kick in and they will be more concerned about you.
* Leave the room and return with ice cream.
* Have a friend call on the phone or have someone "stop by."
* Start to cry.

When you don't know what else to do, simply say, "Let's pray about this." When you can't fix it, change it, or make it go away, in their generation and in ours, what can you do with it? Pray about it. You have to trigger this by saying, "Let's pray about it." Whether you're religious or not, their simple prayer may help you both.

After one of my presentations, a young caregiver went directly back to her community to see the lady who had been crying for days for her mother. She lay down next to her and they prayed together. The lady then fell asleep.

I follow the three "P's": Patience, Practice, and above all, Prayer! —ROBIN MOON, CARING FOR HER HUSBAND

Newfound Spin Cycle

Saturate
Their Obsessions

A person may begin to obsess about a certain task or chore, such as washing their hair, hoarding dishes, or picking at their skin. If they're at the dinner table and are constantly taking other people's cups or plates, give them extra cups and plates when serving. *Saturate their obsessions.*

> *A lady would scream and scream. Caregivers would go in her room and say, "What's wrong? Stop screaming." She would just scream louder. A nutty caregiver went into her room, started screaming, and told the lady, "Scream! Get it all out!" Guess who stopped screaming?*

> *He has gotten to be so fussy about so many things, like wiping spots off the table, stacking a week's worth of newspapers and magazines just right, and polishing, polishing, polishing his silverware before he eats. He can also work for hours and hours on his jumbo-sized word search.* —Marvea

> *A lady wanted to peel potatoes. We got a five gallon bucket and let her peel until her heart was content.*

Some will disagree about letting them use a knife. From my experience, peeling apples or peeling potatoes is a task their body remembers. Because at what age were they taught to use a knife? Very young, so this action is ingrained in them. When I give them knives, the only complaint I've heard is: "This knife isn't sharp enough!" But I'm not suggesting that you leave the knives on the table and leave the room. Maybe boil the potatoes and scrape the skin off with a table knife. If you understand their generation, you will use carrot peelers so nothing is wasted.

Know the person and what their abilities are. And please make every attempt to give back to them what they still can do.

A lady from New Jersey told me how her husband loved to fix the vacuum, but every time he fixed it she had to spend $120 to get it fixed. She hid the vacuum in the closet, which made him more upset because he couldn't find it. I suggested getting extra vacuums from Goodwill or garage sales, then putting one in every room and letting him fix them to his heart's content.

"My dad continually picks at his skin. Any suggestions?" My response: Sleeve socks for arms or long-sleeve shirts buttoned from the inside; or give him something to pick at, like stickers or price tags on items you bought at a thrift store.

Too often, we don't give people the chance to do what they want because we're concerned about their safety or we believe they won't do it right. Don't play out in your mind what you think could happen. Give it a try! Let go of your expectations of how things should happen.

I find that I'm now a victim of obsessive behavior. Whatever I start, I have to finish immediately without any interruptions. An unfinished task preys on my mind until it is done. This is the exact opposite of how I used to be. I used to be exhilarated by having dozens of balls bouncing in the air, so that life didn't become stale. Now I can only concentrate on one thing at a time, and to everyone's distress, I obsess over it until it's completed.

—Excerpt from My Journey into Alzheimer's Disease by Robert Davis

---

The truth is…when we are scared, we want control. —Cynthia

Newfound Saturation

Kick-Starting

At some point the person may lose the ability to start a motion or locate certain parts of their body. "Kick-starting" simply means to start the motion for them.

If a person is sitting down for a meal and not eating, place your hand over their hand and start the motion by assisting with two bites, then let go. Place a comb in their hand. If they look blank, place your hand over their hand and start to comb their hair, then let go. If you ask them to put on their sock but they don't respond, touch their foot and cue them again to put on their sock. It doesn't matter what the task is: If they respond blankly, start the motion and touch that part of their body to get them started. The trick is to then let go.

One of my favorite things is to give everyone lotion and encourage hand massages. When I asked Edith if she would like some lotion, she would nod her head and then just sit there with a dab of lotion on her hand. I put her hands together and helped her rub in the lotion. After a short time she started doing it on her own.

Another way to help the person understand what you want them to do is by demonstrating the motion: You sew one pant leg while they sew the other. You put lotion on one leg, while they put lotion on the other. Your goal is to help the person remain as independent as possible for as long as possible. If the person is struggling, help them today, but let them try again tomorrow. They have good and bad days just like us.

Another possibility is to help the person get dressed but let them finish by having them button their pants or put on their shoes. This helps the person feel like they have gotten themselves dressed.

When Mr. Johnson moved into our community, he was functioning at a pretty high level. He was still able to do some accounting-like work in the afternoon. I took maternity leave for about four months. When I returned, Mr. Johnson was in a wheelchair and had declined rapidly. I asked a staff member what had happened. She said she wasn't sure, but now whenever she asks him to brush his teeth, he just opens his mouth.

Avoid helping too much. If you try to do everything for them, they will become more dependent on you, making it more work in the long run. Allow the person more time to accomplish each task. Then let go.

Morning checklist:
Clothed? Ah, sufficiently.
Keys? Yep just found 'em.
Coffee cup? Full.
Sanity? Sanity?...And we have a runner.

Newfound Start

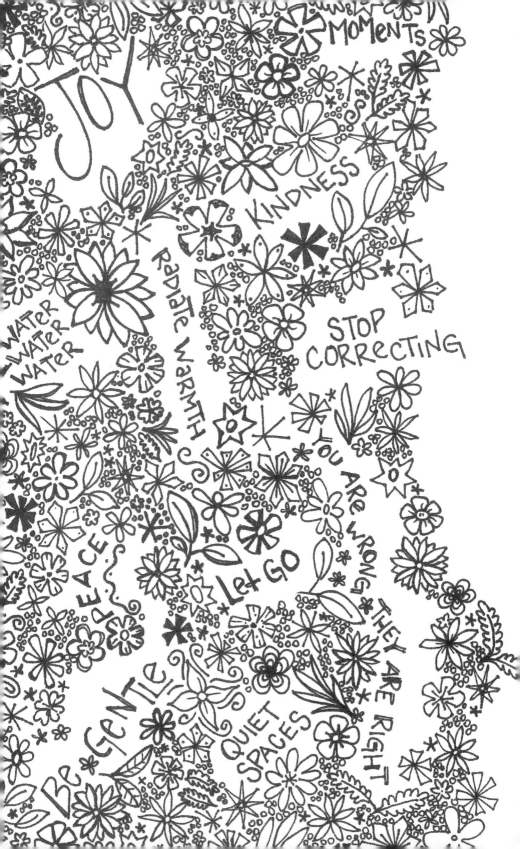

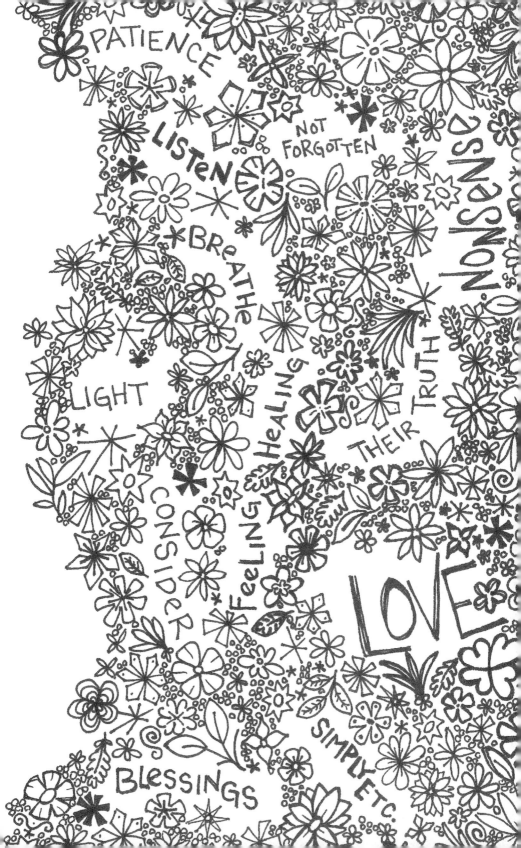

Look Good, Feel Good, Play Good

Can't you tell instantly whether it's going to be a good or bad morning? I could. Every morning I started my program with a beauty hour: curling irons, rouge, lipstick, lots of hairspray, and, of course, Old Spice. My beauty station (a simple chair and end table, where I locked all the supplies) was located outside the dining room. When people finished eating, I invited them over to be beautified. While they waited, I had old magazines to peruse and comfy chairs to sit in. I knew that if I pampered them, even just a little bit, they would look good. If they look good they feel good, and therefore play better.

The clothes they wear also affects their mood. Looking good is recognizing what clothes they feel good in—worn out or clean-cut. What feels good is completely different for each and every person.

Sarah loved to wear red and wore a red cardigan every day. I said to her, "Sarah, I sure like red on you." She replied proudly, "I do, too. My mother never let me wear it because she said it was the devil color, but I like it."

There was a dynamic-looking lady who wore a striking pink dress, pink lipstick, pink rouge, and pink fingernail polish with a white purse and white pumps. Her hair was every bit in place, and she walked with confidence. Because of her short-term memory loss and because this was her favorite dress, she wore it every day. Staff and family didn't like that and had a difficult time getting the dress off to get it washed. Their solution was to pour coffee on it. A horrible solution! Of course, the dress needed to be cleaned every once in awhile, but the answer isn't to damage it or tell the lady that she smells. Think how insulted you would be if someone said that to you. If you think about her personality, and body language, a better answer might be: "There is a handsome man visiting tonight. Let's get freshened up so you will look wonderful tonight."

On the contrary, if the person feels good in pajamas, then let them wear pajamas. It's not about what we think looks good. It's about what *they* think looks and feels good.

> *I received an email from a daughter who was very frustrated because her mother no longer cared about her appearance. Her hair was a mess, she didn't put on makeup anymore, she was untidy, and she would simply sit and rock in her chair all day long. I made a few suggestions and this was the result:*
>
> *"I took your advice and massaged my mom's hands and arms with lotion, I combed her hair, applied a little makeup, and put on one of her necklaces (which she wanted to pay me for). Then she asked where we were going. I took her for a short walk and she was just beaming. I haven't seen her that happy in a long time. You are right! It was my attitude that determined how our visit would go. Thank you for letting me know it's the simple things you do that mean the most and to accept my mom as she is. I cannot change her but I can enjoy her. I can remember the good times with her and smile at the smiles she gives me now."*

Simply start with lotion and go from there. Don't be surprised that when they start to feel good, they will flirt with the maintenance man.

There is no way to happiness; happiness is the way. —THICH NHAT HANH

Newfound Look

Honey, Dearie, Sweetie

How they are with you is how you are with them. If they call you "Sweetie," it gives you permission to call them "Sweetie." If they call you "Ma'am," call them "Sir." If they ask you what your name is, call them by their first name.

I am not from South Carolina, but when I got off the plane there, within fifteen minutes I was called "Sweetie" three times. In utter frustration, I wanted to "bless their heart." Ugh! Whether or not you like to be called Sweetie depends on where you grew up.

For most of his life, Don had been in charge of a manufacturing company. One day he said something needed to be done about these lazy workers. I told him I would get right on it. I didn't get right on it, and he slammed his fist on my desk. I reacted, "Yes, Sir! I will take care of it." After this he became "the boss" or "Sir," and when he made a request we responded with, "I'll get that done, Sir," and would walk out the nearest door. Because of his short-term memory loss we could walk back in within seconds.

If the person is a businessman or school teacher, it's Mr. Evans, Professor, or Mrs. Larsen. This person would probably be offended if you called them Honey. A man or woman of their generation is not "cute." Instead, he is "handsome and charming." She is "elegant and witty."

Staff was given instructions not to call this lady Granny because it was thought to be demeaning. After a thorough discussion, it was apparent that this particular lady responded positively when addressed as Granny. How, then, could calling her Granny be wrong? Everyone has an opinion, but the person's reaction is your teacher.

We were calling our mom Mary, which is the name she went by for many years. But when she was growing up she was called Mary Marjorie. Now she smiles when anyone calls her Mary Marjorie, and I put a big sign on her door with that name. She knows this is her room.

A nutty caregiver shared that she called one of her residents "My Bad Girl." The daughter was in the audience. Growing red in the face, she told us, "Yes, my mom has always been prim and proper, and now she just wants to be the bad girl."

A sister shared that her little brother, who was now 78, was nicknamed Bones. When they were younger they shaved his head and then teased him because he looked like a "bonehead." The name stuck.

I have found that almost everyone has a nickname. What's theirs? What did their friends call them? Because you want to be their friend, it's worth your time to find out.

My nickname is "Mom," but my full name is "Mom Mom Mom Mom Mom …" —UNKNOWN

Newfound Nickname

Men...Being Gentle-men

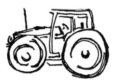

M en need to be needed and wanted, and *they need the illusion of control.* Three things you can say to get a man to want to stay just a little longer: "You are soooo strong," "You are soooo smart," and "You are soooo handsome." (This works with your husband, too. Two extras just in case: "I made supper," and "There is a cold beer in the fridge.")

I think it's funny when we women now think we are going to tell this man what to do. Did women have any authority in their generation? *No.* And now he has thirty women telling him what to do and we wonder why he has "behaviors."

Any chance you get, allow the man to be a gentleman: "Will you get that door for me?" "Would you bring that chair over?" Figure out what this man was good at before he needed your care. What could he fix? What was his occupation? Let him know you still need his help:

* Stacking wood; digging a hole
* Moving a wheelbarrow
* Washing a car (or a van—it takes longer)
* Fixing a radio
* Sanding down a chair to be stained
* Organizing a toolbox (only safe tools, and only real ones—*not plastic*)
* Matching nuts with bolts
* Finding the keys to go with different locks
* Adding numbers
* Counting change in a kid's piggy bank
* Having him report to work (give him a badge)

One day Jennifer, a caregiver, took my grandpa outside to look at her tire because she knew that he used to sell tires. The twenty minutes they spent outside together made my grandpa's day.

However he helps you, say, "Thank you so much!" If he wants to be paid, fake checks are perfect for this. Or give him what you have in your pocket or purse (one dollar bills and change). When he loses that money, someone will be happy finding it later. Men need money in their pocket. Their whole life was tipping the waitress and paying for things. If a man tips you, simply sneak that money back into his pocket later.

There are five things men have had in their pockets for a lifetime: keys, change, a wallet, a pocketknife, and a hankie or comb (the fifth item depends on the man). Now imagine: He no longer has his keys because he can't drive. He no longer has change, and his wallet is empty. Someone took his pocketknife because they thought he might "stab someone." At what age did he get that pocketknife? Probably eight. Who did he get it from? His dad or grandpa. How does he feel checking his pockets and finding it missing? How many times does he check his pockets? Over and over. He's more likely to feel secure here when you put back in his pockets what has been there for a lifetime. Go online and print off twenty dollar bills so his wallet is thick. When you give back his pocketknife, does he stab people? *No!* He puts it in his pocket and brings it out to clean his fingernails. What if he cuts himself? Well, who's more likely to get cut: you or the man who has used it for sixty years? *You.* If you're still concerned, drop a little super glue into the pocketknife. It isn't usually about using it—it's about having it.

How much would it cost to fill the top drawer of the dresser full of red hankies, so he always has one? Not much, but it's a priceless gesture to have many of whatever item gives him security.

I sat down next to a gentleman I didn't know and stated, "You look like a hard worker." He looked back at me. Noticing his attire, I proceeded, "Are you a farmer?" He replied, "Yup." I continued, "Did you have cows?" He answered, "Yup, 'bout twenty-five. I had some chickens too. I even had a blue tractor." I replied, "Wow." He smiled, "Betcha you're wonderin' how I got a blue tractor." I was. "I painted it," he said. We both laughed. He looked at my ball cap and said, "Like your cap." Even though it was my favorite ball cap I offered, "Would you like to try it on?" He nodded, then sat there wearing my ball cap. I asked him, "What's your nickname?" He plainly replied, "Sugar Boy." Surprised, I questioned, "How did you get the name Sugar Boy?" He answered, "My aunt thought I was cute and sweet." The rest of the conversation I called him Sugar Boy, and he smiled every time.

I excused myself and went home for a moment to get six other ball caps to replace the one I had given him. And I put together a bowl of fruit to share. When I returned, I asked staff, "Where's Sugar Boy?" No one knew who I was talking about. Try describing someone with gray hair and glasses in a care community. Eventually, I figured out he was the one yelling from his room. I walked in and said, "Hey, Sugar Boy." Who stopped yelling? "Would you like some fruit?" (He cannot yell and eat at the same time.) "Do you like any of these caps?" He took one and put it on his head, handing me my favorite cap back. I said, "I like that on you." He just winked and nodded as he nibbled. As I was leaving I discovered something else: Other men were interested in my ball caps. I went home with just the ball cap on my head.

Men need their cowboy hat, their John Deere cap, or their fishing cap. I believe that when they're under these caps men feel better. If he has a favorite ball team, have a T-shirt and ball cap handy before you enter his room. He likes anyone who is rooting for the same team. Record his favorite team winning a game and let him watch the game over and over. It feels like his team wins every single time.

If the person was in the military, hone in on their memories; be sensitive to what they may be sensitive to. Tip: To get a military man to stand up, say the Pledge of Allegiance, "Attention!," or "Captain on deck!"

"That shouldn't be out there. That shouldn't be out there. That shouldn't be touching the ground." This gentleman saw a small American flag from the Fourth of July on the ground. He was distraught. I went out, picked it up, and stored it properly. —JOLENE

When any man, military or not, wants to leave, take his arm. There was such a gentleman who thought he had to leave, so I took his arm and asked, "May I walk with you?" As we were walking, he looked over at me and said, "Honey, my bed isn't made." I smiled, "That's okay." (Yes, flirt.) Then I said, "My feet hurt. Do you think we can sit for a bit?" Needing to get back to work, I said, "Give me a moment. I will be right back." People are sometimes shocked at my flirtatiousness, but whose job just got easier because I showed up? *Yours.* This man will wait for me and be the perfect gentleman. Caregivers also get to witness the pure joy that comes over a man's face when I give them a kiss on the cheek or ask to feel their muscles.

An occupational therapist told me that she purposefully wears shirts that show her cleavage. Men are the most cooperative with her.

Go ahead, label the man as sexually inappropriate. Men are men are men are men. When you label him as sexually inappropriate and warn women caregivers not to get too close, does his need go away? *No!* It only gets stronger!

So don't linger in front of him, but do rub his back, kiss him quickly on the cheek, give him a side squeeze, wink at him when you walk by, and even give him a big hug, knowing he will try to sneak his hand up to feel you. HE NEEDS ATTENTION!!! He is a MAN!

For some men, a girlie magazine can be an outlet, and it's familiar from their younger years. I have a scrapbook, so to speak, of pinups. Usually everyone is okay with those—they are safer than Hustler magazine. But there have been times when I brought a copy of Hustler! (P.S., We have to be okay with masturbation. A doctor prescribed Viagra for that very purpose. It worked! The staff could recognize when his anxiety increased and would offer him the Viagra. He took care of business. They protected his dignity and helped with cleanup. He was relaxed and happy again.)

—NATALIE, AN EXPERT IN DEMENTIA CARE

If you don't want to be the flirt, put on a enormous diamond ring and show him you are married. Sometimes that works. If, however, a caregiver or a female resident is being harassed and/or grabbed, someone is clearly getting hurt and a line must be drawn. Switch to a male caregiver, or have anyone who looks older put on a nurse's uniform and become the professional to give him his bath. Yes, this man may simply need to live in all male community, or a Veteran's home. Especially, if a female resident is being physically hurt, there are no exceptions. But if the woman is enjoying his manliness…shut the door.

Picking up what's left, gleaning their manli-hood. —FREDDY

Newfound Gentle-man

Socially Engaged

Research shows that people with Alzheimer's cannot handle large spaces, lots of people, or noise. In memory care communities we take them out of their room into a large space with lots of people and noise because it "looks good" when they are participating. The kids love it when they are socially engaged. Management loves it. Surveyors love it. And we can check it off. "Come on out! We have a sing-along!" "Come on out! We have preschool kids here!" "Come on out! We have an activity!"

When we take them out of their room and into a place with a lot of commotion, they can go into a "blackness." Can they come up to you and say, "I can't handle this situation. Will you take me back to my room?" No. Who's the only one who can see the blackness? We are. Who is the only one who can take them back to their safest, most highest functioning place (possibly their eight-by-ten room)? We are.

Even if the person participated in the church choir their entire life, now with Alzheimer's they may not be able to handle it. But children want to see their parent continue to do the things they have always done because it makes the kids feel better. Ask the child to come to the sing-along and see firsthand their parent's anxious face. Then and only then will they agree to "let it go." It now becomes more important that we sing with them in their room.

When you get to be their age, do you want to "come on out!"? Or do you want to be in your bed, with your blanket and your pillow, and you just want someone to shut the damn door! If you'd choose to simply be comfortable and warm on your last journey, consider that the person you are caring for would like the same thing. But for some reason when someone is in their room too much, we think, "Oh, they are isolating themselves!" Then the kids get concerned and think, "Maybe we should take them to the doctor to see if they are depressed."

Who is creating the insanity? *We are.* We, who want something different than what is happening right now.

A lady expressed, "I am not going out there! They took me to the doctor and now I got these pills, but I am still not going out there!"

Remember, I am not your teacher. Your experience with them in the now is your teacher. Every person is completely different and every day is completely different. One day they may like to sing with everyone, and on another day it exacerbates their confusion.

The ache for home lives in all of us, the safe place where we can go as we are and not be questioned. —MAYA ANGELOU

Newfound Safe Place

Moments
of Discomfort

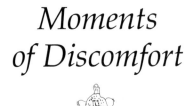

Written by Lori Linton Nelson, expert on pain management.

Pain can often be the cause of irritability, pacing, increased wandering, anxiety, resistance to care activities, and depression-like symptoms. It may be difficult for the person to differentiate pain from another health problem. They do know, however, that they are feeling discomfort.

As caregivers, we often make assumptions by observing a person's behavior and comparing it to their past behavior. Observation and comparison are important, but we must also employ other methods, such as screening tools and simple questioning. Often a person can respond to a pain intensity scale, and caregivers may need to try more than one. Some people may be able to rate their pain on a scale of one to ten, and I know caregivers who find it helpful to show the person a pain intensity scale that uses faces (from smiling to crying), similar to those used in hospitals with children.

Sometimes we just need to help them find the words to describe their pain, such as by asking them whether they "hurt" or "feel bad" in a particular area of their body. And it's important to talk with family about how the person has historically acted when in pain.

Also, it is helpful to review the person's medical history to determine whether there are current or past medical problems that cause them to be in pain now. Arthritis, osteoporosis, chronic back pain, gout, stroke, history of multiple fractures, and diabetes are examples of conditions which can cause both acute and chronic pain.

At times it is so difficult to differentiate pain from other sources of frustration that a caregiver may need to discuss a trial of regularly scheduled pain medication with the health care provider. Most

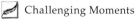

individuals also respond to non-medication–type remedies, such as hot and cold treatments, relaxation, distraction, and massage.

> *Margaret's favorite song to sing over and over again was "Sing a Song of Sixpence." She had nine children, and her joy was to nip off the person's nose who was sitting next to her. Four years had passed since I last visited Margaret. I found her lying on her bed in a fetal position and moaning in slight pain. I laid down next to her and softly sang, "Sing a song of sixpence, a pocket full of rye. Four and twenty blackbirds ..." She whispered, "Baked in a pie." I continued, "When the pie was opened, the birds ..." She whispered, "Began to sing." I continued, "Wasn't that a dainty dish to set before the King." And in the end I nipped off her nose.*
>
> *There was a gentleman who had started hitting the aides. I noticed he was limping, and he told me he was supposed to get his toes amputated. He then asked the aides to take care of me while he took care of business. Later I found out that two of his toes were quite swollen from ingrown toenails. He was hitting because he was in pain.* —SHEILA, A VERY INSIGHTFUL PERSON

If they are completely different today than they were yesterday, it's probably not the disease, but pain!

☼ I've learned that even when I have pains, I don't have to be one. —MAYA ANGELOU

Newfound Relief

Hallucinations

There is a list of things to consider when the person is having hallucinations. Start by looking at their medications; different combinations of medication may cause hallucinations. Check to see if the curtains are closed at night. They might be seeing their reflection in the window and think someone is "peeping in on them." They may have a dream they perceived to be real the night before. Patterns on the walls, chairs, and floors can create hallucinations of spiders, insects, or other little critters. Voices over the intercom are "coming from where?" TVs are also a culprit. (Please refer to the chapter "A Commercial about TV.") Of course the damage to the brain is obviously a large factor, too.

Do not watch commercials, violence, or the news on TV. Get rid of the intercom and walkie-talkie by replacing them with headsets. Close the curtains and avoid anything with patterns. No matter the source, respond to their hallucinations as if they are real. Just saying, "Alice, there aren't any snakes in your bed," won't help. They will call 911 if you aren't going to take care of it. Take action!

Pearl would yell, "There's a fire in the house! There's a fire in the house!" My reaction: "I got everyone out. Let's go." Then we would walk Pearl outside. Sometimes it worked; sometimes it didn't. I wondered if Pearl had ever been in or witnessed a house fire.

Hallucinations are most often visual, but they can also be present through our senses. When they're very real and upsetting to the person, have someone put on a uniform and exterminate what they are seeing. Ask the person, "May I do anything to help?" If the answer is yes, then to the best of your ability do what they want you to do.

When my mom sees someone who's invisible to everyone else in the room, I say "I can't see her, but I'm sure you can. I'll take care of it."

This is honest on our part and yet does not separate you from their experience. Leaving a person who is scared and upset is rarely the right thing to do, so say to them, "Please let me just sit with you till they are gone."

She's still bothered a little by imaginary people telling her not to do this or that. So when she tells me about "him," I tell her that we'll throw him in the river. Then I say, "Of course, Sweetie, the river's still frozen, and he'll go bump, bump, bump on the ice." She asks me, "Is that so?" And I say, "Yep...bump, bump, bump." Then she laughs that beautiful laugh, and we laugh together. —ALAN ROSS, A HUSBAND CARING FOR HIS WIFE

This is a wonderful example of taking the hallucinations lightly, adding a dash of humor. The end result: a moment of joy.

Shut up voices!...Or I'll poke you with a Q-tip again.

Newfound Spiders

Sundowning

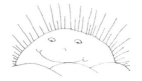

Do you want to hear my theory on Sundowning? They have had it…with all of us!!! They are tired and stressed to the max and have been nice long enough! "It's getting dark. I gotta get home!"

The next time you put the cereal in the refrigerator or milk in the cupboard, drop a dish, or yell at someone, you are *sundowning*. We have simply labeled it for them because they have a disease.

They might need a nap, something "off" happened, they need to get home because kids are getting off the bus, or it's getting dark and Mom must be worried about them. Whatever the reaction, I believe there is a reason.

We know the developmental level of a person with dementia is usually around that of a three-year-old child. What if you took your child to preschool and they didn't have any structure or naps and could run around and do what they wanted to all day? What would their emotions be like when you picked them up in the afternoon? Kids would be crying, kids would be fighting, kids would be sleeping in corners, kids would be clinging to the only adult, saying, "Where's my mom? I want to go home."

Does this remind you of any other environment? Yes. A memory care community without structure and routine.

To reduce sundowning have at least five things that happen every day to create structure and routine:

1. Beauty hour. Which caregiver or person in the family enjoys doing hair? Every morning take time to make them look good because when they look good they feel good.
2. Walking, walking, walking. Sun. Fresh air.

3. Napping. Fatigue is a major cause of confusion. Who has a calm disposition and can put people to sleep by reading a dull book while yawning? Or simply consider: What puts people to sleep? Church service. Church service.

4. Sing during shift change. If they see coming and going they will want to go, too. Whoever loves to sing, start singing fifteen minutes before shift change, away from the exit, and sing until second shift is in place.

5. Lawrence Welk, a baseball game, an old western, a polka dance show after supper. It is difficult for them to ground themselves, so we need someone who just wants to put up their feet and relax. Wrap people up in blankets, put their slippers on, and help them to relax by relaxing yourself.

Here is the routine I created, but please create your own:

8:30	Beauty hour	2:00	Upbeat activity
9:30	Exercise	2:30	Coffee
10:00	Coffee	3:00	Relaxing activity
10:30	Walk/bingo	3:30	Rest
11:30	Devotion	4:00	Activity depending on the mood
11:45	Relaxing music	5:00	Dinner
12:00	Lunch	6:00	Ballgame, western, or musical
1:00	Nap/quiet reading	7:00	Relaxing activity

There is meat and there is gravy. The meat of the day (five things) never change, but whatever happens in between is gravy—it all depends on their mood.

People with dementia don't operate by a thought process. They operate by how they feel. —JOLENE

Newfound Routine

Wandering, Hoarding, Combative

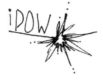

We have the ability to create whatever *perception* we want with words. When I say, "She has been wandering all morning. We've got to get her to sit down," how do you feel about what she is doing right now—positive or negative? *Negative.* When I say, "June is ninety-six and probably walked a mile this morning. We'd better get some vodka glasses and shoot water together," how do you feel about what she is doing? *Positive.*

When I say, "That lady is hoarding stuff in her room and we are going to clean it out at lunchtime," how do you feel about what she is doing? Negative. When I say, "Margaret feels more secure when she is surrounded by sugar packets, apples, napkins, and silverware. I am glad she feels secure here." Positive.

When I say, "John is combative," how do you feel about him? However, when I say, "John felt threatened by what I just did," who has to change?

The language we use defines how everyone feels about what the person is doing right now. If I can challenge you to do one thing, it is to change the language you use. How do you think society feels when they hear about Alzheimer's and connect it with words like *combative, agitated, exit seekers, violent,* and *sundowning?* Even the phrase "patient with behaviors" alters the perception to "these people are scary." For those of us who have cared for people with Alzheimer's, are they scary monsters? Absolutely not—at least not until we show up and correct them or test them.

They can also sense your intention. One day I didn't want to be there and I came in with an agenda. When I pulled out my normal bag of tricks, this man looked me in the eye and said angrily, "You don't care! You don't care!" In that moment he was absolutely correct, and he could sense what I was trying to hide. People with Alzheimer's are truth tellers, and when they respond negatively to you, you might want to look in the mirror. We are part of the equation and we create outcomes.

On the flip side, families can have an unrealistic expectation of wanting their loved one to have "peace of mind" and blame caregivers when the person is upset. This disease is scary, period. No matter our every effort, they will still have many moments of confusion and fear.

> *A daughter in tears told me how she called to see how her mom was doing. The lady on the other end of the phone checked her charts and said, "Your mom was combative today."*

How would you feel if I said to you, "Your mom was combative today"? Don't question your mom; question the people giving her care.

In health care systems, we like to label people and blame their actions on their disease. When we do this we are forgetting the most important question: *Why?* Why are they behaving this way? When you walk out a door today you aren't labeled an "elopement risk." But when you get dementia, you will be considered an elopement risk and will probably be medicated for your agitation.

Take the challenge: Change your language, which will change your perception, which might change the way we *all* view people with Alzheimer's.

 What goes into the mind comes out in a life.

Newfound Language

Age Appropriate

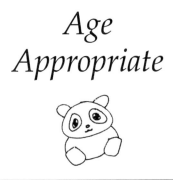

If I read you a nursery rhyme your grandmother had read to you, how many of you would feel better almost immediately? *That's not age appropriate!* If I gave you a big teddy bear to cuddle with, how many of you would cuddle? *That's not age appropriate!* If I gave you a brand new coloring book and colors, *how many of you would color right now?*

Who are we to decide what is age appropriate? If the person is content or engaged, then savor the moment. A steady beat, like a lullaby or a nursery rhyme, will slow down their heart rate. "The three little kittens, they lost their..." See, you can't help but say "mittens."

> *When I was first redesigning dementia communities, I would walk in and insist that the stuffed animals had to go. I was going to make this place "look beautiful," and stuffed animals were not part of the equation. I wish I would have paused to observe how stuffed animals brought comfort. I was young and inexperienced, and it became about me and how the place would look. Today it isn't about me or looking good. All decisions are based on bringing comfort to those who live here.* —JOLENE

> *My friend wished very much for her mother to say her name, Virginia. During a care conference, a staff person told her that her mother carries around a doll whom she calls "Ginny." This was the ultimate gift—to know that her mom was holding her!*

A doll will become real to them. When this happens, treat the doll as real: "Let me take care of Ginny while you eat." "I'll take care of Ginny tonight. You get some rest." "Shhh...Ginny's taking a nap." There might be moments when the person is aware that the doll is not real. Make it no big deal and simply say, "Oh, I guess it is a doll. It looks so real."

Take heed: Do not have just one doll or one stuffed animal because there will be more than one person for whom it will provide comfort. And if the doll loses its arm, fix it immediately.

Bonus: When children visit they get to interact with our older generation. Keep a box filled with coloring books and old toys. Nothing delights me more than seeing a child coloring with an older person, and nothing is more fun than coloring with a child.

Growing old is mandatory, but growing up is optional. —WALT DISNEY

Newfound Toys

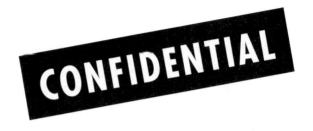

Too often, care communities focus on confidentiality. "You know that man with Alzheimer's in 313? Can I say his name?" What do we lose in the process? We lose the person and their identity.

I challenge you to take the toughest person you have—the one yelling from his room, the one pacing, or the one who falls out of her wheelchair repeatedly—and write down ten to twenty things that anyone has done to make this person feel better. One community went back and applied this to the lady who had to use the bathroom every twenty minutes. I am sure you have no one like this in your community, but I like to share the story anyway. ☺

They wrote down what made this lady feel better:

"Good morning, Sunshine!"

"Barb, you have such rosy cheeks!"

"Barb, I love it when you wear pink." (She wore pink every day.)

"Barb, would you like some English tea, no sugar?"

Talk about her brother Bob: "Bob sure looked out for you." "Bob is a wonderful big brother." "Bob let you ride the horse while he walked."

"Barb, I am so jealous of your naturally curly hair."

"Barb, be nice to those men today."

Whisper in her ear, "That girl can be so bossy."

Bring her ginger cookies.

"Your husband, Harland, is handsome. You got quite the catch."

When Barb asks, "Where's my husband?," say, "He is at the shop."

"Barb, would you like a back rub?"

"Hi, Sassy Pants."

They made copies of this list and shared it with everyone: housekeeping, maintenance, staff, and families. Everyone was asked to do one thing on the list during every shift. What need do you think went away? The need to use the bathroom. When they need to use the bathroom every twenty minutes, what are they seeking? *Attention.* When they are yelling, what are they seeking? *Attention.* When they are pacing, what are they seeking? *Attention.* When you tell them they have beautiful rosy cheeks, what are you giving them? *Attention.* When you sneak something or whisper something, what are you giving them? *Attention.*

Then I hear there is not enough time for that extra task. Okay…take them to the bathroom every twenty minutes. How long does that take? Twenty minutes, every twenty minutes! Which would you rather do: take her to the bathroom, or tell her she has beautiful rosy cheeks?

Frontline caregivers are drilled on confidentiality: "We can't post this information in places where everyone can see." The fact that they have naturally curly hair, love English tea, or their brother took care of them—is that a confidentiality problem? *No.* But caregivers think it is, because that is what the community focuses on. Yes, medical information and a bowel movement this morning…confidential. But allow the ones who give the care to share with everyone, including families, what works with each person, because they are the ones with the answers.

Then we put everything in the care plan. When the person asks, "Where's my mom?," do you think the new caregiver is going to say, "Hang on a minute, let me check your care plan"? No one has time to check a care plan. Even if they did, where would that information be in the care plan? Furthermore, caregivers would rather work shorthanded than work with new caregivers who don't have answers. These answers, the ones we find that make someone feel better in the moment, are stronger than any medication. Allow caregivers to tell everyone.

How do families feel when they visit if they don't have the answers? One person says to them, "I want to go home." The next person asks, "Have you seen my son?" The next person states, "You have to get us out of here. They're locking us in here!" Then their dad asks about his wife, who is no longer living. How does it make families feel when they don't have the answers? Helpless. Uncomfortable. Anxious. Guilty. "I can't believe I left my dad here."

Then the person will ask the question they ask fifty times a day: "Where are my kids?" The visitor responds with, "Well, Shirley lives in Alabama, and Richard moved to Connecticut, but I bet your daughter Sally will take you out to lunch on Tuesday." "TUESDAY?!? I am not staying here until Tuesday! Somebody find my kids!!!" Do you think this visitor is going to want to come back?

The greatest gift we can give is to teach everyone how to visit, which means giving everyone the answers. To begin this process, put a blank sheet of paper behind everyone's door. When anyone finds an answer that makes the person feel better, they write it down. Then when you have compiled many answers, rewrite them on a bookmark, which can be slipped into a little pocket next to each person's door. The new caregiver or a new visitor can respond to questions with, "Let me check on it," and have a place to easily find the answers.

Smart memory care communities have a binder at the main entrance with a page for each resident. On each page is a list of at least ten things that make that person feel better, plus the answers to the question they ask fifty times a day.

What if I jabbed the person on the shoulder and said, "Hey, Stink Pot!" Most likely management would say, "You can't call him Stink Pot!" Is Management my teacher? NO!!! Is the State my teacher? NO!!! The only person who is my teacher is the gentleman who smiles when I jab him and call him Stink Pot!

When you do something a little edgy, like swear with them or let someone walk around without shoes, you need to have it written into the care plan. Understand that when the State walks in, they only see a small picture of what is happening. If what's happening is questionable, they want to look at the care plan and see why you did what you did, and how it creates quality of life for this person.

Put in the care plan that this person falls less when they are not wearing shoes. Put in the care plan that, "Harold calms down when you swear with him," or "Bill takes a bath when you give him whiskey (apple juice warmed up in the microwave) before, during, and after his bath."

If you were cited by State for doing what is best for this person, you would have been cited for something either way. It tells me this individual from State doesn't understand dementia. There are no hard rules, and anyone who creates rules around people creates the insanity. Each person is different. But let me be clear: State is not your enemy. We need State to ensure that people are being well taken care of and have quality of life. When State does a survey, show them where you are struggling. Inquire whether they have any ideas.

My point is this: Many caregivers are working with the fear of getting in trouble: "What if State walks in when I'm swearing?" "What if Management walks in when I call him Stink Pot?" "What if I get into trouble for doing this?" My advice to caregivers: Don't ask for permission—ask for forgiveness if it doesn't work. The one who holds the magic wand (answers) is the one who is giving the care. Caregivers know this person better than their own family members do. Give caregivers permission to make mistakes, and give them kudos when they create a moment of joy.

When you, nutty caregivers, look for answers, please do not play out in your head whether or not something will work. Your head is not your teacher. The only person who can teach you what works and doesn't work is the person in this moment, so try everything. What worked five minutes ago might not work five minutes from now. This is why this person, in this moment, is your only teacher.

When anyone catches someone creating a moment of joy, write it on a piece of paper and post it for all to see. *Thank you! Thank you for caring with love, kindness, and a large dose of nuttiness!* Nutty caregivers are the best! Acknowledge them!

You're mad. Bonkers. Off your head... But I'll tell you a secret... All of the best people are. —LEWIS CARROLL, *ALICE IN WONDERLAND*

Newfound Bonkers

Let's Talk about Sex

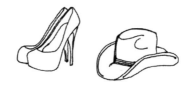

Written with Linda Larkin and Natalie Kunkel.

With dementia the real issue is not that they are "intimate," but who they are "intimate" with. Children still think, "Mom is a virgin," no matter how many kids she has. But interestingly enough, they are proud of their dad because, "He's still got it."

In dementia settings, sex is so buttoned up that we don't talk about it, and we certainly don't have policies to deal with it. There are so many issues that come into play: What will their children think? How will someone handle their spouse being interested in another? What about that guy hitting on that other guy? Lordy. We have created the problem, not the people enjoying it.

Sex is a basic human need and function. It is included in Maslow's Hierarchy of Needs. Would you deny someone food or shelter? Sex is a need so innate, it doesn't go away when the brain begins to fail. When we take care of our loved ones with dementia, we must understand that just because they don't know how to verbally express their need for intimacy or need to be touched, doesn't mean they won't show you. Sometimes it's in ways we're not prepared to deal with. Especially if it is a prominent member of the community making sexual advances or a person found masturbating. Let me remind you: God made us sexual beings. Who are we to judge?

Part of the reason this subject is so hard to get our arms around is that there are so many people bringing their own feelings and experiences to the table. We have different generations and cultures with different understandings of what intimacy is and what is considered appropriate.

In most settings, if it doesn't harm someone else then why are we trying to stop it? It's understandable that we don't want to see two people engaged in sexual activity in common areas, but in the privacy of their own room, why not? There is nothing more powerful than feeling wanted and needed. That is a feeling most folks with dementia just don't get enough of. When you think about it…if you're constantly being corrected, told no, and kept apart from someone you want to spend time with, it effects your self-esteem, your sense of self-worth, and your outlook on your own quality of life.

It's incumbent upon us to enable these encounters when possible, and it's possible more times than it is not. Caregivers who are compassionate, empowered, and creative can make this possible for those who want to find a part of themselves that has been lost.

What's most important at the end of the day is the way the people involved feel. Just to be touched, held, caressed…this is a wonderful feeling that they may not have experienced in a long time. What a gift to have that back, at a time when so many abilities are fading.

A wife said it so beautifully: "I know I cannot be with my husband twenty-four hours a day. I'm glad he feels loved when I am not there."

At a conference a lady shared that now when she visits her husband he is always sitting very close to another woman. And then she added, "I was always sitting close to him. When we were together, we were close to each other. He simply needs to be close to someone, even if that someone isn't me." She worked through it herself. It was an honor to witness.

When Elmer and Helen became a couple, the families did not condone the two being alone in a room. We never told the couple they couldn't be alone, but when we saw them disappear behind the door, we grabbed our cleaning bucket and vacuum and knocked on the door: "Housekeeping!" One day Elmer said to a caregiver, "You have the worst timing." They never felt wrong, dirty, or forbidden, and we were successful in disrupting the experience disallowed by the family. They kissed and held hands and spent their days together.

—NATALIE

A lady was asking what she should do because her husband was holding another woman's hand. I gently looked into her eyes and said, "He is holding your hand. He is holding your hand." It clicked, and she said, "Oh…well he does call her Betty, and that is my name." I reminded her again gently, "He still loves you Betty. He still loves you."

Personally—and I realize it shouldn't be personal—I am more unsettled when a husband is cognitively well and expects his wife to have sex with him even if she doesn't know who he is.

One of the most difficult days is when the spouse realizes they are visiting as a visitor, not as a spouse.

Each couple is unique; each situation is unique. Focus on how each person responds. You can tell when an intimate moment is causing pain and confusion as opposed to when it is causing pleasure and relief. Never forget that we all need to be needed, loved, and touched. Sex is less about the act and more about the "feeling." We all love feeling loved, no matter how old we get. If no one is getting hurt…shut the door. It's a good feeling, not an affair.

Oh, I'm sorry. I didn't know you had the authority
to judge me…Is Jesus hiring???

Newfound Intimacy

Traumatic Moments

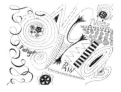

Trauma in the present moment will escalate the dementia: someone they love dies, they take long trip, they're admitted to the hospital, or they experience earthly trauma such as a hurricane, fire, or tornado. These extreme forces of stress and strain can drop them into a place of no return.

There are traumatic memories too: being molested, witnessing a murder, time spent in war, losing a baby, near drowning, racism, being a survivor of the Holocaust, and so forth. These traumas resurface with dementia, and the person may feel like it's happening right now.

A wife shared that when her husband was nine he had asked his mom for a baby brother. Unfortunately she died while giving birth, and still to this day he blames himself for her death. Because of his dementia, his feelings are as strong now as they were when he was a child.

Painful memories are not forgotten, even in dementia. Respond as though whatever it is, is happening right now. Give the person space to feel their pain. Comfort them by saying, "I am so sorry this happened to you." It is in the reliving of the story that the person is often able to come to terms with whatever pain or hurt is buried, especially deep hurts.

My mom wasn't a pleasant person when I was growing up. Anger was always below the surface. When her disease progressed, she shared in bits and pieces that her uncle had touched her button and she was not to tell anyone. My anger toward her dissolved, and compassion seeped in. Alzheimer's healed my mom's pain and our relationship.

We all have pain and bitterness we have not dealt with. Just know that it will come out with dementia, and that can be a blessing. This disease doesn't allow us to stuff our pain any longer. When it resurfaces, it's an opportunity to heal what hurts.

If this person grew up in a racist environment, those emotions and inappropriate language are going to come back up. There is no way of stopping it, and one has to understand that it is not personal. It may be directed at you, but it's not about you. It's their own issue, their own anger.

Maybe the person needs forgiveness for the trauma they have caused someone. Whatever the situation, there is no better time than now.

> A woman came up to me and said, "My mom is mean to me when I visit, saying that I am spoiled, and Daddy's favorite." I asked her, "What do you think that's about?" She replied, "Well, Dad and I have always been close, and I think my mom has always been jealous." I simply suggested, "You might want to ask forgiveness."

For those of you who don't yet have dementia, I would like you to consider something: Do you have built up anger? Do you have unresolved issues? Do you still harbor great pain from a memory? If so, now is the time to heal to find the greatest peace possible.

Anger repressed can poison a relationship as surely as the cruelest words. —JOYCE BROTHERS

Newfound Resolve

Violent Moments

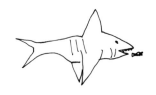

Written by Randall Bruins, RN, who specializes in forensic psychology.

Compassion is the path to building rapport. Rapport is the best defense against being attacked and the best resource for defusing aggression. Having a connection with our fellow humans is what we all long for. The neurotransmitter dopamine is produced when we feel connected to others, giving us a sense of wellness and ease.

Managing my own emotions and gaining their trust are often the biggest challenges. Desperation is what escalates violent behavior. If I think about what has helped me overcome an exasperated frame of mind, it would be someone listening to my despair and offering empathy to my situation.

What comes to mind is an experience I had with a Vietnam War vet. He had PTSD (post-traumatic stress disorder) from his war days and at times would react to his environment with excessive frustration that could escalate to violence. Getting to him before he became violent was the key. John could be seen with a very serious look on his face, not making eye contact, pacing, then heading for his room and pacing again. One day while pacing he started yelling, making threats and gesturing to the people around him—scaring them. So I started pacing with him. He didn't object. I didn't ask him what was bothering him; instead, we just paced. It didn't take long before he disclosed how angry he was at "Connie." She'd promised him an outing but the trip was called off. John told me that it was because Connie didn't like him and was punishing him. I responded in a tone of voice that was similar in intensity to John's: "When that happens to me, I too can get very unset." We arrived at a place where we could sit and talk about how hard it is to not get to go on an outing. And as we developed a rapport, he accepted my offer to talk with Connie to find out when the next outing was scheduled and report back to him.

John was able to calm down. I followed through to help resolve the problem, gaining John's trust. And from that experience John gained a resource in someone whom he believed would help him get his needs and wants met. Don't most of us need others to help us out of a bad state of mind from time to time? It's a gift to have someone understand our pain. This is where it starts.

When I see a person as being unduly upset over a seemingly minor offense, in order to build rapport I will escalate my own emotional response to match theirs, validating what they're experiencing. Bonding takes place, and then I can begin to de-escalate myself emotionally while remaining connected to the person. Frequently the person will follow me into a calmer emotional state. This is an example of extending true compassion toward a person with whom it can be difficult to feel generous. It's just so much easier to condemn someone for their behavior and then retreat to the safety of our own superiority. But that is not the way we help someone who can't connect effectively with others. They are just like us: they want connection and intimacy. But the world just doesn't want to give it to them.

Jolene's two cents: If a person becomes angry, fights, or yells for you to leave, do it! Honor their request. Stop the confrontation and leave. Return five minutes later with a different approach, or send a different caregiver, and see if you get a better reaction.

A gentleman had a tendency to hit when staff cared for him. A nutty caregiver, who was quite small, put her hair in pigtails, spoke like a child, and said with a hug, "Good morning, Grandpa!" She became the person he would not hit—a child.

Where fear is present wisdom cannot be. —Lucious C. Lactantius

---

Newfound Compassion

I don't want him to... *The doctor says...*

My sister says... *They don't think...*

We can't... *The state says...*

He shouldn't... *Management says...*

I want my mom to...

W hose journey is this? "Here is your [handful of] medication." "No, Dad, they don't allow smoking here." "No, sit down. You might fall." "You can't stay in your bed all day." (If you stay in bed, they think you're depressed and will take you to the doctor for antidepressants.)

We can do it...we can keep you safe and healthy for five more years! Five more years you get to live with Alzheimer's. "No, you already had three bowls of ice cream." "No, you're a diabetic, you can't have dessert." (Why did we create insulin?) "You must eat so you stay healthy." Believe me, we can keep you "safe" and "healthy."

Or...would you rather live for three months, eat what you want to eat, sleep when you want to sleep, walk when you want to walk, have the right to fall, and die with two cookies in your mouth because you are a diabetic? If you want quality of life instead of quantity, consider that the person you're caring for would like that, too.

I just found out my mom has cancer. I am oddly grateful. Now she doesn't have to live with Alzheimer's for the next ten years.

The right to sleep

"How do I stop my mom from hitting me when I wake her up to change her?" Let her sleep. Her reaction: "What if she has skin breakdown?" I replied, "We can talk about 'what if,' but let's talk about what is happening right now. Right now does she have skin breakdown?" "No." There's no perfect answer, only the better answer. Is it more important that she sleeps or more important to wake her up to change her? Answer: getting her sleep.

"What if he..." "What if they..." "What if...We'd better not..." "I don't think we should...What if..." Replace with...What IS.

The right to be warm

Do you know how much unnecessary anxiety they are experiencing simply because they are cold? *Colder than cold.* How thick is their skin? Paper thin. How is their circulation? Poor. You may be sweating, but they're still cold. When I see a person wearing three sweaters and a coat, I think, "Yee-haw! They got themselves warm!"

> *In a care community I noticed a lady sitting at the table, shaking. I sat next to her and she repeated, "I'm floored. I'm floored." Putting my arm around her to console her, I said, "Let's get you wrapped up." Thinking I would take her back to her room to get her warm, I asked the nurse, "Where is her room?" She replied, "Oh, she needs to sit there because we need to monitor her."*

Are we having them monitored (watched) to the point that we have taken away the one thing we can give: warmth and comfort? This is their last journey on this earth. This is the one thing we can give them! Do we really need to monitor people this way? Even if she does have to sit there, get her in a comfy chair and wrap her up. A hat, a scarf, fuzzy mittens, cozy socks, a warm blanket, a hot water bottle, or something simply to hold. We have all of these things. And yet…And yet…

The right to fall

> *When I visited a care community, there was a lady sitting all alone in the middle of the dining room with a pained expression on her face. I bent down and put my hand on her knee. She said, "Daddy, Daddy." I asked, "Is your daddy a big man?" With a blank stare she replied, "I'm a good girl. I'm a good girl. Daddy loves me." This lady believed she was being punished, because the med aid said she needed to sit there as she was a fall risk.*

As a human being, we have the right to fall. No one wants anyone to fall but it will happen, even if you are standing next to a person. Here are some solutions I've seen communities implement:

* Placing a fall leaf outside the doors of residents who are a fall risk. Every staff person knew they needed to be checked on twenty times per shift, not just once.
* Installing silent motion sensors above beds. A staff person was quietly notified on their pager when anyone was moving around.
* Having a policy stating that people have the right to fall.

The right to refuse medication
When you are dispensing medications and they close their mouth, they are telling you *No*. It is abuse to shove pills into their mouth against their will.

The right to refuse a bath
No one has died because they didn't get a bath.

The right to peace and quiet
Wander guards—an alarm goes off every time they use a door they shouldn't be going through. Motion guards—when they move in their bed or their chair, an alarm goes off to let everyone know. *Alarms are not okay!!!* Evacuating the care community with loud fire alarms is insane! We can change the sound and do these drills without the use of a piercing noise.

The right to choose
When I moved to Montana I saw an ad in the paper for "Smoking Assistants." The community was hiring people to smoke with people. Brilliant!!! You want that job!

A scotch, or a cigarette, may enhance this moment more. Are we keeping them so safe that we have taken their life away? This is their home; consider that we are supporting systems and not the people who live here.

The right to eat
Families don't like it when the person eats too much and gains weight in the early stages. "Keep them healthy," we say. Consider they need all of this weight gain because as the disease progresses they will become skin and bones. How many people have you seen pass away overweight with Alzheimer's? Doesn't happen.

The right to sweets
A lady began to tear up. I asked, "What's going on?" She said, "My husband was a diabetic, and my daughter, who is an occupational therapist, insisted he shouldn't be eating desserts because...what if he goes blind, what if he loses a foot, etc. Every meal my husband ate in another room because he would get upset when he saw others having dessert when he couldn't. I wish I would have insisted that he get his dessert."

When it's your last journey on this earth, do you want everyone else deciding what you can and cannot have? Notice how easy it is to take things away from someone else. But what if someone took away the things you want?

When we do what everyone else wants, it gets pretty muddy. When we do what this person wants, it gets pretty clear. Crystal clear. It does not take words for this person to show you what they want. Listen…listen…listen with all of your senses. Listen to this person.

Sometimes the hardest thing and the right thing are the same. —THE FRAY

Newfound Rights

Taking Them to
the Doctor?

Why are we continuing to take them to the doctor? Maybe we are thinking that if we just get the right combination of medication they will get better. Or we want to know what stage of the disease they are in. Or perhaps we want to know what to expect in the future. All of these things just foster an illusion of control, when in reality there is none. There currently is no cure for Alzheimer's, and the medications that are prescribed for it have side effects that often make it more difficult for the caregiver to care for the person. And if the person is prescribed heavy psychotropic medications, we essentially lose the person, making it impossible to maintain a viable relationship with them.

Is it really important to figure out what stage of the disease they are in? Even if you figured out what stage they are in, what difference would it make? Every day things change, and everyone with this disease goes through it differently. The only thing that is predictable is that it's unpredictable. Trying to figure out where the person is at in the disease and what to expect next is the insanity. The only certainty is that the disease will progress.

An eighty-two-year-old woman proclaims, "My doctor says I have Alzheimer's. I've learned to beat and fight everything in my life. I don't know how to fight this." You could see the weight of the diagnosis. If she could remember that someone told her she had Alzheimer's, I question the diagnosis and wonder, is it really necessary to add more weight at the age of eighty-two, when she could simply age as she will age?

My uncle was diagnosed with a rare brain disease. It has been slowing his communication and brain functioning for many years. Now the doctors came back and added that it was stage seven Alzheimer's. What would be the point to adding another uncontrollable diagnosis for my aunt to stress over?

A better question is this: What's happening right now when you take the person to the doctor to try to figure out this disease? Or, what happens to the person's mood when we insist every day that they must take their medication? The stress level goes up, and when the stress level goes up, where does the functioning go? Down. Who suffers the repercussions? Everyone! Has anything changed? Only your hope that what if ..., which is a rightful hope. But at what cost?

Are there times when they will need to go to the doctor? Of course: if the person is physically hurt, in pain, becoming aggressive, having severe anxiety, mania, or depression, or isn't sleeping at night, which directly affects the caregiver. But aside from when it's absolutely necessary, avoid the stress on the person and the waste of time and money.

Consider what people of their generation do to make themselves feel better: a hot toddy, a cigarette, a nap, a drive, a walk, a good cry, a hot water bottle, Vicks VapoRub. The remedies are endless and the effects are priceless.

She stood in the storm and when the wind did not blow her way, she adjusted her sails. —E. E. CUMMINGS

Newfound Remedy

Medication

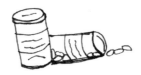

Written with professionals in the medical field.

There is still no cure for Alzheimer's. There are medications prescribed in the treatment of the disease, but from my experience of listening to caregivers and family members, the only certainty seems to be uncertainty with regard to how well, if at all, the medications specific to Alzheimer's are working. Some caregivers and family members say they seem to notice a difference, while others say they only notice the unpleasant side effects. When the person experiences extreme anxiousness in the early stages, there are non–Alzheimer's-specific medications (such as antidepressants, sleep medications, and pain medications) that are sometimes prescribed which do have positive effects.

Alzheimer's is very unpredictable, varying from day to day and from person to person. The medications specifically prescribed now for Alzheimer's are designed to treat the symptoms in the *early stages* but have not shown to be effective in the middle to late stages. These medications are not a fix—they at best stall the inevitable. Determining how effective these medications are is difficult because of the unpredictability of the disease.

The bottom line is this: The least amount of medication is best. First figure out other ways to help them cope. You, or some other reliable person, need to become well informed on any medication prescribed. This means first asking a doctor about it (what it is supposed to do, what the side effects are, how effective it is supposed to be, and so forth). Then ask a pharmacist about it, as they often know more about the specific medication than the prescribing doctor does. And finally, do some research on the medication. Becoming fully informed enables you to make a sound decision as to whether this specific medication should be taken, or a different one should be prescribed, or if it's best to refuse all medications. No matter how much research you do, the person's response is the real teacher.

There is a line that can really only be determined by the person with the disease, and it needs to be determined early on while their reasoning abilities are still fully functional. That is, whether or not they want to be medicated, and if so, whether there is a point at which the medication should be stopped. Some people may refuse medication altogether, like some terminal cancer patients do, but others may want to be medicated to the very end in the hopes of some miracle cure. In either case, it is something that should be discussed and decided on as soon as the person has an idea of what they're dealing with. To ignore the issue, thus leaving it up to the caregiver and family members to decide later on, is asking for conflict. Family members seldom agree on anything.

All of the preceding depends upon action: getting a diagnosis as soon as possible, becoming fully informed, and making the hard decisions up front.

Initially, our family firmly believed meds were the only answer. After I researched the antipsychotics and other medications "usually" prescribed to manage agitated behavior, it worried me because of their potentially dangerous side effects and their propensity to sedate.

Mom had severe sundowning: crying, agitation, anger, nonstop questions, repeatedly phoning people to get answers, etc. She would get up eight to ten times a night—walking the house, angry, cursing and throwing things, and wanting to leave to go home.

When we stopped fighting with her, decided it was okay to fib to her, and changed how we treated her, we saw changes. The techniques in this book work, and seeing is believing: Our family finally started to be "believers" in modifying our behavior to improve hers.

While modifying our behaviors, we considered melatonin, too. Since it is a hormone that our bodies produce, it seemed like a safe option for her. It's been about three months since she has been on melatonin and four months since modifying our behaviors (we're getting pretty good at therapeutic fibbing now!). The change is nothing short of miraculous. Thank you. She is so much more "our mom" again. —Marge

It seemed to make my aunts, who lived in another state, feel better when Grandma started taking Alzheimer's medication. But I could see it wasn't making Grandma feel better. —A granddaughter caring for Grandma

There are many factors that need to be considered when dosing and administering medications to elderly patients in general, especially those who suffer from memory loss or some kind of dementia. Often times, clinical staff within a facility will call and ask for a stat fill on a PRN medication such as Ativan to address behaviors they are experiencing with a resident with dementia. When asked by pharmacy staff to describe what triggered the behavior, clinical staff are often at a loss for such information. Because of the many demands for their skills and talents, short-staffing, and the many other residents to care for, clinical staff are often tempted to put a temporary bandage on the issue and also fail to plumb the depths of what the resident is feeling or experiencing—the root cause of their pain, whether it be emotional, physical, or both. This short-term solution of PRN medications, while a temporary fix at times (but not always), can play into a much bigger problem or increasing behaviors that are stressful to the resident, family, and staff alike.

I received a call from a gentleman who was caring for his wife. She was a former schoolteacher and loved small children: they made her come alive in an animated way. I could hear the desperation in his voice as he explained how his wife had attempted to physically harm their nine-year-old granddaughter. We went over the long list of possible triggers, ruling out any source of physical pain such as a toothache or an ear infection. He then perked up and said, "She hasn't had her toenails clipped in a couple of years and they are starting to curl over her toes. Maybe that's causing her some pain." I suggested he have their daughters take their mother to the foot doctor for a "pedicure." A week or two went by. He informed me that they had not had any issues since. —MINDY

There are numerous factors that need to be looked at before the person is given a "magic pill." Also, realize that when medication isn't taken regularly, it can actually be toxic.

It was a big concern and worry whether our friend with Alzheimer's, who lives alone, was taking her meds and refilling her prescriptions. One time she had an antibiotic medicine that she was to take over five days. After two days the meds were all gone. So I worked with the doctor and we called the pharmacy. They offer a free program where they package the meds in little bubbles for breakfast, lunch, dinner, and nighttime with the date. Then you can see if they are taking the correct medicine. It was also easy for her to read the information that reminded her about what she is taking. They even delivered it for free. She resisted this in the beginning because she wanted to stay with her old routine, but it was too hard. After three days of fighting me on this, she finally gave in. Being a nurse, she did not want to give up and admit that she couldn't keep it straight. —KAREN, A FRIEND

I have seen over and over again when people go into hospice care and we slowly take them off their medications and give them choices, they get better. Living longer with more lucidity. —A HOSPICE NURSE

Keep in mind that it is not our place to get the person healthy; meaning, we shouldn't medicate the person based upon our hopes or make them adhere to lifestyle choices we want. What do they want? Do they want quality of life or quantity of life? They're going to decline and pass away—it is the natural order of things. Until there is a definite medication that cures, consider letting this process happen naturally. Their generation was not a generation of "pill poppers." Yes, when our generation gets there, we will want our vodka and our medication. But this is their journey. What do they want?

And in the end, it's not the years in your life that count. It's the life in your years. —ABRAHAM LINCOLN

Newfound Quality of Life

Transitioning Moments

Don't wait for the roses.
Stop and smell the daisies. —Jolene

When Is It
Time to Move?

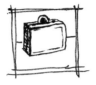

This is a very common question, and my first reaction is, "How is the one who is giving care?" The most common reason people move is because the caregiver/spouse ends up in the hospital, or dies, and now the family has to quickly make decisions about where to move the person. The family had no idea the dementia was this bad; two people can cover for each other quite well. The person with Alzheimer's is then moved quickly without preparation. Please, please prepare. Prepare for a move even though no one is ready or willing. Regularly check in to see how the caregiver is doing. Look at their health and well-being first because they are the ones who are suffering. If you ask, "How are you?," they will say, "I am fine." "Fine" is not an emotion. If you don't want to lose two people to this disease, at some point it becomes no choice.

And yet, to separate a couple will break the spirit of both because they are essentially lost without each other. If one is bound to the other and determined to love and care for this person till death do they part, then it may be an honorable decision. As long as no one is getting hurt. I have heard horrific stories of spousal abuse and I have heard heart-wrenching stories of love.

Women caring for men: The man becoming physically aggressive is one of the main reasons women concede to giving up care. He no longer has the ability to control his emotions/reactions. So when he gets angry or frustrated his way of responding is by hitting or yelling.

Men caring for women: Incontinence is the main reasons men move their wives. Typically men have been not caregivers. They aren't biologically built to be the nurturer. In the caregiving role they believe, as they always have, that they can "fix it." Insisting that she can still make meals as she always has, keep the house clean as she always has, and serve him as she always has. But she cannot.

Abuse is common due to fatigue and extreme frustration. Men also tend to be in denial longer, leaving their wife at home while they go to work. The wife then calls fifty times a day, which speaks to the point she is afraid to be alone. Another sign that it is time to move.

Daughters caregiving for parents: Often daughters think, "How can I move them out of their home? I am the world's worst daughter." Many feel guilty about this decision. Guilt? How does it help? You, as a daughter, are making the best decision in this moment. Give up the guilt. Pause…be honest with what you believe is the best choice. There is no best choice, just the better choice. Expect it to be difficult. Moving someone is simply difficult. But consider they might be nicer to nutty caregivers than they are to you. I've often seen them function better around complete strangers.

Children tend to wait and wait and wait until they get permission from their parent. No one is going to say, "You'd better have someone else take care of me. I am ready to move." At some point families must make the tough decision and expect it to be difficult. It may only take days to adjust or it may take months. They usually adjust. This, too, shall pass.

Will the person function best in a home they have lived in for forty years? Yes, essentially, if they still know where they are. However, they could walk out their front door and think they have just been visiting. Others suggest that it is best if they have time to adapt to a new home before they decline. Both are valid.

If the person lives alone and they have left the stove on or wandered off and gotten lost, or if they simply call you fifty times a day, it is time for them to move. It's best to come up with a reason they would understand for moving, and tell them that it's temporary. It's less threatening when it's temporary, even though you know it is probably permanent. "It's just for the winter." "The doctor says for a couple of months, till things get back on track."

A son literally went on his mom's roof and tore it apart so she could see that she needed to move while the roof was under construction. Another family told their mom, "The pipes are frozen," and shut off her water. Another used the excuse of a bug infestation. This may not seem okay to you, but the perfect answer does not exist if the person is adamant about not leaving their home. These are reasons the person would understand, so it makes the move easier.

It was a blessing when my mom broke her ankle because she had to move into a care community. Seeing her brace helped her to understand that she needed care. We didn't take the brace off until she had adjusted to the new place, even though her ankle was long healed.

To ease the transition for both the person with Alzheimer's and the spouse, start with respite care in small increments. This way the person gets used to being around other people and the spouse gets used to taking care of themselves. It is extremely difficult for a spouse to go from 24/7 caregiving to nothing. Be sure to ask the spouse which part of caregiving brings them joy, such as sharing meals or putting the person to bed, so that they are still a part of the journey if they choose to be.

I have seen many spouses move the person they love into a community because they simply cannot do it any longer. When they start to feel better, they insist on taking them back home, only to find that it is beyond their ability, again. It is very difficult for them to accept that they cannot.

The doctor said, "I know you don't like the idea of moving. But your wife and I are worried about you. We are not doing this to punish you. What is happening right now is not your fault. We love you and are trying to do what is best." Affirm their feelings. Affirm that it is not their fault. Affirm your love.

When is it time to move? I honestly don't know. In a perfect world you would want to live with them for a month, and what you see would tell you the answer, but they have to let you in the door first.

Please do not move the person over and over. Two months with you, two months with your brother...Your intention is honorable, but the constant change does not benefit this person. Moving them from community to community because you are not happy for one reason or another isn't the answer either.

Whenever a new resident moves into our community, it is not the resident who needs reassuring—it is the family member who has to walk away who needs the love. I am the one who stays behind to comfort them as they leave.

Even the big, strong, stable men stop in to get a long hug and encouragement that their loved one will be safe and cared for. They are fragile. Giving up the care of your loved one is not giving up on them. —René Draiggers, LPN

At some point you must make a decision. You cannot predict the outcome. You simply know that what is happening right now is not working. Then you walk step-by-step. And, yes, they will want to go home. But even if you take them home, they will still want to go home. Home is a feeling, and with Alzheimer's, home is another place and time. Give them a reason they understand to move. Then give them a reason to stay wherever they are staying, just a little longer.

Emma moved into our community from the East Coast. She didn't have kids, and it was her nephew and power of attorney who made her move to the West Coast. She clearly didn't have Alzheimer's. She walked ten blocks one day with me because she wanted to leave! She was mad because she had thought she was just visiting her nephew, but he left her here. I never met her nephew. He didn't visit. I still think of Emma today. She may have been old, but this was not okay.

Just because you're in a stressful situation doesn't mean you have to get stressed out. You may be in the storm. The key is, don't let the storm get in you. —Joel Olsteen

---

Newfound Home

Choosing a
Care Community

The community should be memory care specific. Families will move a person with dementia into assisted living because it looks "normal" and no one has to admit they have Alzheimer's. Now they have fifty people who make them feel like something is wrong. The person will be ostracized and bullied and will isolate themselves in their room because they can't handle it. So then the person has to be moved again in six months because the way they're behaving is "not appropriate."

I am often asked, "How can we help our independent residents understand those with Alzheimer's?" It can be done, but it's nearly impossible to get an elderly person to change the way they react to someone coming in and out of their room. One possibility is to give the cognitively well person something to give the "wanderer" or "shopper," like a box of Kleenex, a newspaper, a scarf, or a cookie. But it's more important to choose a community that's memory care specific because people with dementia function at a higher level when they are with other people with dementia. The person is thinking, "I'm doing pretty good. These people are crazy."

Too often families place their loved one in a beautiful, expensive building because it "looks good" and makes them "feel better." But for the person with dementia it's hard to relax because everything looks grandiose, like a hotel. Look for a memory care community that looks like a "lived in home" and supports the person, not your ego.

Memory care is a different world, a different environment, and a different way of being with people. It's not about the building; it's about the people who work inside the building. Are they kind? Are they attentive? Are they smiling? Do they understand Alzheimer's? Do they know the history of each person they are caring for?

When I began as a CNA twenty-nine years ago, I had no idea what lay ahead for me. But soon, I was transformed into a person caring for people with all types of personalities. I would never exchange my time for another job. My children mentioned several times, "Mom, why don't you find a real job." I would simply tell them, "I have one." They said this because I got up each day between 3 a.m. and 4 a.m. and worked every other weekend and every other holiday. They saw how tired I was. So why did I love my job so much? Because I received love back threefold; that still lives in my heart to this day. These were truly "loved ones"—parents, grandparents, people we should be kind to and treat with respect.

Here is one of my many stories. One morning at 5 a.m. it was time to get Anna up. I helped with her morning cares: her personal hygiene, getting dressed, and making her bed. She was sitting up on the side of her bed, and I was bent down, trying to put on her shoes. Suddenly, Anna leaned over, put both arms around my back, and gave me a big hug. "You are the best family I have ever had." Tears welled up in my eyes. I got up, hugged her, and told her I loved her with a smile. Yes! My beloved family, I have the right job.

—FROM THE LOVING HEART OF ROSEMARY BRACKEY

I have seen rural communities who give great care because it's simply a community inside a community. The caregiver knows this person because they were their neighbor, their waitress, or their student. There is no greater gift than to be known.

The ideal memory care community has eight to fifteen people, with two caregivers and a full-time activities director, in a homelike setting: residential kitchen, small living room, and small dining room. I have seen houses in residential areas that have been remodeled to be memory care specific. What a great concept!

There are benefits to a memory care community being on an "aging in place" campus, especially for couples. This allows them to stay together because the spouse maintains his or her well-being in independent living, while the person with Alzheimer's is participating in memory care.

It's also ideal when memory care communities can support different levels of care: one neighborhood for the early stage with people who are walking, walking, walking (wandering), another for the middle and late stages. The question to ask is: "As they progress, will they be able to stay here?" Nothing can replace caregivers knowing this person from beginning to end.

Overall this is a complicated subject and there's no one answer. You know how in the good ol' days there were only three flavors of ice cream: chocolate, vanilla, and strawberry. Now we have thousands of flavors. It's the same with health care. We used to have three flavors: retirement, assisted living, and nursing home. Now we're creating more and more flavors because we know the baby boomers will not accept only three flavors. My advice: Pay attention to how you feel when you visit different communities. Ask yourself: Is this a community that takes care of its employees? If the employees are taken care of, the person will be taken care of, too.

Things to look for in a memory care community

* Full-time activities director for no more than twenty people. This is the "fun" person who creates lightness, silliness, and sweetness. Hire the personality, not the degree.

Mary, our fabulous activities director, takes residents on golf cart rides, flies kites, takes them fishing, and has horse races complete with mint juleps.

* TV is not the focal point. When I see people sitting around a fifty-six inch TV in the middle of an activity room...red light! When TV is the babysitter, it insinuates that people have nothing to contribute—no value or purpose—which is far from the truth.
* The caregivers are wearing regular, brightly colored clothes. In memory care, people aren't aware that they have an illness. They don't know why they are here; therefore, they are more comfortable with friends than with people who are trying to "take care them."

I don't typically wear bright colors as I am a little fluffy. But I noticed that their eyes light up when I wear bright scarves and clothing. Now I wear something colorful every day because it's these little things that matter the most to them. Little things that matter: scratching their back, a smile, and remembering not to ask, "How are you doing?" —RENÉ DRAIGGERS, LPN

* It looks like a place where they can relax, move about freely, and be exactly as they are. Memory care is a social model, not a medical model, of care. The person with dementia reacts to people and what they see in the environment.
* The flooring has few transitions and is not patterned.

* It has rocking chairs. Rocking relaxes both the mind and the body.
* People are sitting in chairs they brought from home. Wherever this person gravitates to—the quiet space, the busy space, or their room—is where their chair (their place of comfort) should be. If their chair is visible to them, they're more likely to find comfort here.
* The decorations are from the 1940s to the 1970s. It's not about making things "beautiful" by today's standards, it's about triggering memories. Look for walls filled with wedding photos and pictures of local churches, war memorabilia, movie stars from their generation, farm animals, fish to catch in the area, and pictures of the residents in second grade (we're all cute when we are little).
* There are spaces where they can go shopping, hold a baby, work on a workbench, or create art.
* Outside there are birdhouses, a shed, a doghouse (no need for a dog), a screened-in porch, a path with benches along the way that lean slightly forward so they are easy to get in and out of, a clothesline with sheets blowing in the wind, bunnies, chickens (or at least statues of animals that look real), the country's flag, a windmill, or anything that you would find in your own backyard.
* Curtains that pull shut instead of blinds because people cannot operate blinds, and blinds cause agitation.

This a good place to start when choosing a community. Nothing is perfect. Stop the search if that's what you're looking for, but thank God there are many, many communities today that provide quality care in an environment designed specifically to support those who have Alzheimer's.

I repeat…look for a community specifically designed for memory care—not a community that just looks good or, the opposite, one that has an institutional look. The day we see a bar for happy hour, slot machines, and we're hiring people to smoke with residents, we will have arrived at the understanding that supporting a person is more important than supporting a system. Get ready…marijuana is right around the corner.

Home is the place we love best and grumble the most. —BILLY SUNDAY

Newfound Community

What to Expect

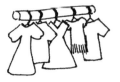

Expect other people to be wearing your mom's clothes. The sweaters you brought yesterday created a moment of joy for everyone.

Expect everything to get lost. Anything you bring in is a donation. Do not expect the caregivers to locate the one item you brought.

Expect hearing aids, glasses, dentures, and diamond rings to get lost. It's a losing battle to continue to replace these expensive items.

Expect "shopping." People will rummage through each other's drawers and closets. Let it go! Better yet, give them a shopping bag and let them shop.

Expect others to be in your dad's room. Twenty residents have twenty rooms because they don't know which is theirs. Allow everyone the freedom to wander and explore their home.

Expect people to be taking naps everywhere. This entire space is their home and they need their naps.

Expect someone to walk out of a room completely naked. Life is happening here, which in my opinion is better than medicated dullness.

Expect people to say exactly what they are thinking. They will tell you that you have a fat ass, but they will also compliment you on your dress.

Expect gossiping, bickering, swearing, a bit of chaos, and one-liners when you least expect them.

Expect smiles and hugs from people you don't know.

Expect dancing, singing, and everyone (including caregivers) being a little "off."

Expect two people to be having a lovely conversation no one understands. It's just nonsense. ☺

Expect it to be a messy. People live here.

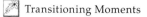

Expect not to see a calendar of daily activities. Activities will happen moment by moment.

Expect caregivers to be wearing regular, colorful, everyday clothes, not scrubs.

Expect that when you ask them, "What have you done this morning?," they will say, "Nothing." That's why we take pictures. To show the joyful moments...they forgot they had.

And most of all...**Expect** to be appalled, to be warmed, to be scared, to be silly, to be confused, to be smiling, to be sad, and to be loved. This place and the people in it will become family. The majority of caregivers love what they do and particularly love people with dementia. If this place truly understands Alzheimer's, expect this place to allow everyone to be as they are.

So...expect the unexpected. Suffering happens when you expect something different than what Is.

Appreciate each moment as an unrepeatable... unpredictable miracle. —Sister Mary Rita, S.P.

Newfound Expectations

Creating a Safe Haven

I f someone took your treasures, would you still find pleasure being in your home? Being surrounded by what you love is what makes it home.

Before you move the person into a new home, first take a picture of their place of comfort, their greatness, and where they sleep. Pick up those three places and drop them down as closely as you can into the place they are moving to. You think you will remember where everything belongs, but in the last minute you will move things around so it "looks good." Moving their things around only heightens their confusion.

Moving is difficult, whether you have dementia or not. To ease the adjustment, I strongly recommend moving everything prior to their arrival. Have the favorite grandchild take the person out for lunch, to a park, or on a country drive. Do not involve the person in the decision making. The goal is to reduce the stress that comes from moving.

What can you put in their room to let everyone know who they are (their greatness)—a picture they painted, a portrait of their family when the kids were little, a souvenir from a place they frequently visited, perhaps a collection? The trick is to place their treasures in a similar location to make the new room look like home.

A gentleman who was a doctor has copies of his diplomas hanging on the wall and is still referred to as Doc.

Place of comfort

Where is their place of comfort—a sofa in the garage, the kitchen table, their sewing desk, a recliner in the living room? If the place of comfort is their recliner, what side is the end table on? Right-hand side? Then the end table needs to stay on the right-hand side. *Do not* buy a new chair.

When it isn't their chair, they won't find comfort in their new home.

A lady wanted to bring her mom's favorite swivel rocking chair, but the community wouldn't allow it because of the fall risk. Make every effort to move their place of comfort, even if it swivels.

A lady brought in her chair with an ottoman. A nurse came in and tripped over the ottoman. It was considered a fall hazard and was removed. I ask you, who's more likely to trip on the ottoman? The nurse or the person who has had it for thirty years?

A lady was sharing how she hadn't moved in yet. She was moved in except for her favorite chair.

Their greatness
What is their greatness and where would they look for it? If they like to read, where do they look for their books? Under their pillow? Then put their books under their pillow and not on a bookshelf. If you put their sewing supplies in a plastic container and put it in the closet, are they going to know where to find it? *No.* The sewing bag needs to be on the left-hand side of the chair, where it has always been.

Where do they sleep?
What kind of pillows do they like, how many, and where are they located? How many blankets? Which blanket is their favorite? What has always been on the bedside table?

Where is the lamp? Which side of the bed do they get out of? Do they sleep on their back, side, or tummy? Do they wear socks to bed? Are their sheets tucked in? If you change even one thing, like buy them a new comforter, this is no longer "their bed."

My mom wouldn't sleep in her bed. I bought her a new purple comforter to replace the old purple one. My mom didn't start sleeping in her bed until I placed her orange and green afghan at the end of it, where it had always been.

A lady remodeled her three-car garage to look exactly like the first floor of her father's house. The paint on the wall was the same. The coat was still hanging behind the door. The bathroom was in the same location. The old recliner was there with the end table on the right-hand side. "We moved my dad to another state and he didn't even know he had moved." Where does his level of independence stay? The same.

If you want to have them live with you, I highly recommend that you move your things into storage and make your home look like theirs.

Side note: We all know that moving into a smaller space presents challenges. What do you keep and what do you pass along to family? Instead of selling the person's belongings at a garage sale, donate the stuff to a care community. I'll bet the belongings they've collected over the years will bring joy to many. Or…they can be sold at a community yard sale to raise money to purchase a piano or an old-style hairdryer, so the world can go away for the many women who live here.

We cannot give them their memory back, but we can give them an experience that triggers memory. —Moyra Jones

---

Newfound Haven

"Where's My Room?"

It is very difficult for people to find their room, and rightfully so, because the doors all look alike. Have you ever noticed in retirement communities how people have distinct decorations outside their doors? Most people are able to figure out ways to distinguish their doors. However, people with dementia usually do not have this ability. So it's even more relevant that we create as many clues as possible:

* Hang something they love that's uniquely theirs next to their door: a cuckoo clock, a painting, their graduation picture, etc.
* If he flies airplanes, hang a picture of his plane.
* Place the person's signature about four feet up at their eye level. (Some people recognize their signature far into the disease.)
* Where does the person think they are? Apartment? What number? Write that number on their door.
* Put the person's old door, with their door knocker or doorbell, in the new place.
* What color was their door? Paint it that color.
* Hang a sign with the name of the street they lived on.
* Did they have a beloved pet? Put a picture of that pet next to their door. (Be sure to ask what they see in a picture before you hang it, because they may see something completely different than you do.)

A lady I was visiting loved roses, and outside her room was a picture of a lovely red rose. I complimented her on the picture and she said, "I don't like that. It's a mule's butt pointing right at me."

Following is an example of a door decoration of someone who enjoys fishing.

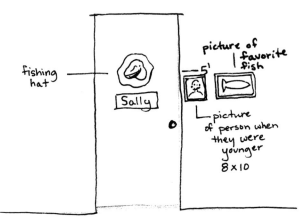

Pat loved to fish in her younger years, and that was something to be proud of in her day. She had a picture of herself holding a thirty-pound salmon on a dock. This picture was hung right outside her room. When anyone entered the community, she would show them the picture and talk about how big the fish was. When Pat could no longer communicate very well, she would point at the picture and nod her head; her eyes showed you how proud she was of that day.

If the person doesn't have family, ask caregivers to decorate the outside of their door. We want everyone who walks by to see a person, not the disease.

We too often love things and use people, when we should be using things and loving people. —Unknown

---

Newfound Door

Playing Favorites

What are their favorites? Favorite drink? Favorite snack? Favorite ice cream? Favorite sweater? Favorite place to sit? Favorite person? Favorite tease? Favorite blanket? Favorite place to visit? Favorite subject? Favorite music?

When you find anything that causes a positive reaction, write it down and share it with everyone! Avoid writing general statements like, "My mom loves to talk about her brother." Write down specific statements such as, "Bob, your brother, is quite a fisherman."

Emily's Favorite Things

* Buttered popcorn with lots of salt.
* Call her "Em."
* Chocolate milk.
* Point out her painting of "Starry Night" by Van Gogh on her wall.
* Em is a poet. Read one of her poems.
* Feed the birds together, or turn on the baby monitor so she can hear the birds.
* Notice her picture of her little brother, Gill, and her older brother, Bob, on the end table.
* Say, "Em, you have gorgeous blue eyes."
* Say, "Hey, Ornery!" (it creates a smile).
* Sing "Catch a Falling Star" or "His Eye Is on the Sparrow"
* Read funny short stories from *Reader's Digest*. Her favorites are marked.
* Likes to sleep in a cool room with lots of blankets.
* Soft serve ice cream (any ice cream flavor, but not sherbet).
* Let her wear her favorite blue nightie all day.
* Prefers walking barefoot.

Share this list with everyone! Write down their evening routine and put it on the wall next to their bed; write down their morning routine and tape it to the bathroom mirror. So when you leave for a much needed vacation, the routine can still happen because you wrote it down.

The greatest gift you can give is to write down who this person is so that other people can provide the care and you have space to take care of yourself.

My favorite thing is when people remember little things I told them. Like seriously? You actually listened to me? Thank you. —UNKNOWN

Newfound Favorites

Remember
Their Greatness

What has brought this person great joy throughout life? Softball is one of my great joys. I also have four brothers, so any man who thought a girl couldn't play, I took them on and took them down!

To create a moment of joy for me when I get dementia, simply say, "You're an awesome softball player!" I'll smile. Then point to any man and say, "I bet you I could kick his butt," because in my family we talk trash: "I'm gonna kick your butt, Mama." "Gonna take you down boy."

The glove I want and need is the one that stinks up my car and will probably stink up my room. You're going to want to throw away my glove or Febreze my glove, and I hope I am able say, "It's not about you. My room…my glove!"

My glove is the same as their chair. After sitting in the same chair for thirty years, what does it start to look like? Not so good. What does it start to smell like? Really not so good. But it's not about you—it's about what brings this person comfort. Clean it and accept that it simply won't ever "look good." But amen, it brings comfort.

My glove is the same as their outfit. It has a few holes and may smell, but they like it so let them wear it.

I also love to play cards. I could play cards 24/7 if someone would just let me. I love the game 500. When I get dementia I may not be able to play a perfect game. But if you correct my game, would that create a moment of joy for me? *No!!!* If you beat me, would that create a moment of joy for me? *No!!!* If my man beats me twice—game over—and he gets nothing at the end of the day!

Let go of your expectations of how they should play, and let them feel like they win every time.

A gentleman pointed out that his wife loved to play cards. However, if he simply asked her, "Would you like to play cards?," she would not respond.

170

But if he took the cards out of his pocket, she would take them from him and deal them out. "You let her win, didn't you?," I asked. "She plays a perfect game, as she always has, and beats me every time," he replied.

My grandpa and I loved to play board games. Now I have to practice patience as he has three of a kind in Yahtzee and fills in a large straight. It has become hilarious as we laugh and make new moments to be cherished.

—TAYLOR LAVENDAR

Often in the early stages they stop "doing their greatness" because it creates frustration; they can't do it the way they always have and they know it. In the middle stages they are less aware of their losses, so get to the good stuff like this granddaughter did:

When my grandfather was starting to show more moderate signs of dementia, some of our family members grieved the loss of our ability to participate in our most meaningful shared experiences with him: playing gin rummy, fishing, golfing, and accompanying him to church services. What we found was that success and joy were still possible when we skipped right to the good stuff in these experiences. To do that, we boiled each activity down to the parts that were the most enjoyable for Grandpa and then re-created those.

Instead of being bound by rules and score keeping, we focused on what he could still do and what he still wanted to do. The good stuff for him when playing cards was holding the cards in his hand, moving them around on the table, sometimes sorting them, and always having carrot sticks, celery, chips, and his favorite Gorgonzola dip. We sat around the table and laughed and snacked, and it didn't matter if our idea of card play met anyone else's expectations because it worked for us! When it came to fishing, we took Grandpa on a drive near the water to smell the salt air, practiced casting in the backyard, sorted hookless lures in his tackle box, looked at old pictures of his biggest catches, and then had fish for lunch. We didn't have to clean the boat or stop at the marina to refuel it, and no more gutting and cleaning fish. This was nice! Skipping right to the good stuff definitely has its rewards.

We used this same method to bring him the fellowship of church through our hugs, and we lifted his spirits through listening to his favorite hymns and reading his favorite Bible passages. His golfing became walks amid the smell of fresh cut grass, putting practice with brightly colored golf balls, and a ride in the golf cart with a little breeze on his check. Before going home, he would order the same lunch at the golf course restaurant: a club sandwich and bowl of soup.

Once we gave ourselves permission to get to the good stuff, our time with him became much more meaningful and less stressful. He no longer felt the pressure to perform tasks or steps in a specific way, and we got to revel in the joy of the doing without worry about completing whatever we were doing together.

P.S., This "get to the good stuff" lesson also carried over into our own lives. Every once in a while we might just make cake batter and stop short of baking, cooling, frosting, slicing, and serving the cake because we decided to just lick the spoon and call it a day instead! So go ahead…get right to whatever the good stuff is in life. It's okay!

—Mara Botonis, Bill's granddaughter, author of *When Caring Takes Courage*

Simplify, simplify, simplify, so they can still do what they are really good at.

Can't make a dress *but can* pull out a hem
Can't fix a car *but can* clean a car part
Can't make a meal *but can* snap beans
Can't make a bed *but can* stuff pillowcases
Can't go fishing alone *but can* go with you
Can't remember birthdays *but can* sign cards
Can't make apple crisp *but can* peel apples
Can't drive a car but *can ride* with you
Can't "go out to eat" *but can* eat at friend's house
Focus on what they *can do*

Every pitch is a new game. —To Taylor, Love Mom

Newfound Greatness

Habits of a Lifetime

One of my habits of a lifetime is sleeping with my feather pillow. My niece Stacie has to brush her teeth before bed and have a glass of water on the bedside table.

When someone has Alzheimer's, it is very difficult for them to tell us what their habits of a lifetime are, so while they are still at home, and while they can still communicate, observe them. What sets them off and what calms them down? Write it down!

There was a belligerent man who was in assisted living, still very cognitive but very uncooperative. I knocked and entered his room at about 9 p.m. The room was very warm, he was resting on top of his covers with his day clothes on, and there were pictures of horses all over. I explained that I was just visiting and asked him about the pictures. He told me he was a Texas Ranger and rode all over the United States to compete in rodeos. We had a delightful conversation about him sleeping under the stars and being a bachelor all of his life while roaming the countryside. When I left the room, I thought, "He sleeps on top of his covers with his clothes on because he is accustomed to sleeping under the stars, and his room is really warm because he is used to the heat living in Texas." If he were not surrounded by pictures of horses, he would essentially lose his sense of identity. I now understood pieces of him, and why he had been uncooperative. He's never been married, but now he has thirty women telling him what to do. This was an opportunity to write down his habits of a lifetime. Imagine how aggressive he would be if he had Alzheimer's and we tried to put him in pajamas and tuck him into bed.

She may be Catholic, but the real value is that she carries a rosary in her purse. He was a farmer, but what's important is that he got up at sunrise and went to bed at sunset. She is an avid reader and reads every night at 7:00 p.m. in bed with a pillow under her knees, two pillows behind her back, and a glass of wine. The details make all the difference!

Here are some "habits of a lifetime" people have shared with me:

* Three walnuts before going to bed. At Christmastime I stock up.
* Three firm pillows: one between his legs, one between his arms, and one at his head (positioned just right). He slept on this right side.
* A certain pair of socks on her feet to go to sleep. She and her husband went camping and she forgot her socks. Her husband drove forty-five minutes out of the way to buy her a specific brand. *(Where did she find that man?)*
* A bar of soap at her feet between the mattress and sheet to fall asleep. Yes, this is a true story. I thought she might be crazy until I shared her story with others and discovered that more than one person claims it relieves leg cramps.
* A spoonful of peanut butter every night before bedtime.
* Another lady had to have the window cracked open, even in the wintertime. The person next to her said she checked her windows before going to bed to make sure they were closed tightly and locked.
* A daughter lit up: "Now I know why my mom doesn't eat breakfast here! It's because she has always had a cheese sandwich with hot water for breakfast."

We are all made so beautifully different—no two people are the same! And who is going to think to serve a cheese sandwich with hot water for breakfast? Not me. We are all just around the corner, or maybe a few corners, from needing someone to care for us. If you write down your habits of a lifetime, you are more likely to get the kind of care you want and need.

The less we interfere with a person's lifestyle, the easier it is for them to adapt to new surroundings. —CHAPLAIN R. A. WILCOX

Newfound Habits

Personal Questionnaire

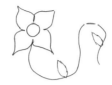

1. *Name:* Emma Smith
   Maiden name: Bradley
   Prefers to be called: Em
2. *Name of person filling out form:* Julie
   Relationship: Daughter
3. *Do they ask for their spouse but do not recognize them?* Asks for Bill, her husband, but he is no longer living.
4. *Do they look for their children but do not recognize them?* Knows me but sometimes doesn't recognize my siblings when they visit.
5. *Do they look for their mom?* No
6. *Do they perceive themselves as younger?* Yes
   If yes, please describe: I believe she thinks she is in her thirties because she looks for Bill and doesn't always recognize us as her kids.
7. *Describe the "home" they are looking for (e.g., ranch, small town, farm, city):* In her thirties she lived in Warrensburg, Missouri. So talk about humidity, small town life, big blue house with large front porch and swing, barn dances at Stevensville.
8. *Describe the person's personality prior to onset of disease (outgoing, introverted, etc.):* Very social and polite in public but in our house she was always busy and the boss…she wants it her way. Very much bossed my dad around. If she asks you to do something say, "Okay, I will get right on that," but just leave the room so she "thinks" you are taking care of it.
9. *Describe the changes you see with dementia:* Frequently swears, which she rarely did before. She can no longer handle a social function. Gets anxious when she isn't doing something, so keep her busy or on a routine.

10. *What makes the person feel valued (e.g., talents, occupation, accomplishments, family, hobbies)?* Very proud of her baking. She made the best pastries. She makes sure everyone has had enough to eat. She'll do household tasks like laundry and dishes but doesn't like it.

11. *What items are significant (familiar) to them (e.g., favorite chair, sewing box, jewelry, furniture pieces, tools, purse, wallet, keys, hat, family pictures, heirlooms) and what is the story behind each item?* Doesn't go anywhere without her purse, but frequently misplaces her purse, so we spend hours looking for it. I will bring you ten purses. She has a favorite recipe book, doesn't wear jewelry, likes lotion and her favorite orange comfy chair.

12. *What is their exact morning routine?* Usually gets up around 5:30, but stays in her pajamas till 8:00 a.m. Give her coffee and kitchen tasks when she wakes up. Drinks five or six cups of coffee with cream but no sugar. Likes a big bowl of Honey Nut Cheerios and a spit bath with a hot wet washcloth. Likes to putz around while picking up. Coffee always in her hand.

13. *What is their exact evening routine (bedtime, snacks, specific night wear, grooming, how they relax)?* Goes to bed around 9:00 p.m., has a martini (we will supply the glasses and vodka), no socks on her feet, and bed sheets not tucked in (messy room). Feather pillow, glass of water (no ice), and Danielle Steele books under her bed. Sleeps in the nude and in the wintertime lots of blankets.

14. *Clothing preference (e.g., dresses, shoes, color of clothing, hats):* Colorful relaxed-fitting dresses, prefers being barefoot unless she is "going out," no bra.

15. *Preferred beverage:* Martini, or water in a glass (no plastic and no ice); coffee with cream and no sugar.

16. *Favorite snacks:* Anything sweet or salty, ice cream, cookies, popcorn with lots of salt and butter, peanuts in the shell.

17. *Favorite meal:* Mashed potatoes, gravy, corn, fried chicken.

18. *What would they get "cleaned up" for (e.g., church, outing, friends coming over)?* Going out with friends, or a good-looking man.

19. *How did they get washed up, or when you were little how did they give you a bath (morning or night, soap brand, washcloth, sponge bath, tub or shower, privacy)?* Sponge bath, Lava bar of soap, hot wet washcloth, eight towels so she is constantly covered up—very private. Doesn't like to be rushed. Needs the feeling of control.

20. *What are their "habits of a lifetime" (daily activities, housework they enjoy, nap time, usual eating times, smoking, drinking, walking, working, etc.)?* Coffee in the morning. Takes a ten-minute nap after lunch and walks every day (we will hire someone to walk with her). Has to be busy so ask her to help with sweeping, wiping tables, preparing veggies or fruit (we will bring veggies from the garden), and arranging flowers.

21. *List significant interests throughout their life (hobbies, recreational, intellectual, job related, such as sewing, cooking, raking, fishing, gardening):*
    Ages 8 to 20: Oldest child, so helped her mom take care of siblings, making sure they were looked after, cooking, cleaning.
    Ages 20 to 40: Housewife with four kids, cooking, walking, loved her flower garden (pink roses and lilacs were her favorites). Involved in 4-H. Took her own flowers to fair. Organized social functions.

22. *Religious background (religious affiliation, prayer time, significant spiritual symbols, traditions, favorite verses, attending church):* Attended Lutheran church—knows all the old hymns. "His Eye Is on the Sparrow" is a favorite.

23. *Cultural background:* Strong German upbringing.

24. *Favorite music:* Frank Sinatra, Doris Day, Perry Como. I will copy her favorite CDs and bring in her stereo.

25. *Favorite TV programs:* PBS documentaries, Lawrence Welk.

26. *Favorite movies/musicals: Singing in the Rain, Anne of Green Gables.*

27. *Can they tell the difference between someone on TV and a real person?* Sometimes she yells, "Get these people out of my house!," and no one is there but the TV is on.

28. *Talents:* Singing, dancing, and gardening. Always humming or singing when doing housework. She will dance with any man who asks since my dad didn't dance. Hasn't done gardening work for years, but waters my artificial plants.

29. *Please describe marital status and if they were married more than once:* Married once, but will bring up her first boyfriend, "Whip."

30. *Spouse's name:* William—called him Bill unless she was mad at him.

31. *Describe distinct characteristics of spouse (e.g., funny, hardworking, beautiful, smart):* My dad liked to play cards. He was smart but

would rather play than work. They often fought when he played poker and drank.

32. *Where was the spouse when he/she was at home (e.g., working in the field, attending church, working in the kitchen, going uptown)?* Worked late at hardware store or was playing cards.

33. *Number of children, names, and type of relationship:* Four
Terry: Oldest boy; listens to him.
Lisa: Oldest daughter; most likely to fight with.
Julie: I just agree with my mom. I don't like to rock the boat.
Greg: Youngest boy; her favorite, I think because he reminds her of her little brother, Gill.

34. *Who might they be worried about or ask for?* Greg. Who she sometimes thinks is Gill.

35. *What would that person be doing during the day (e.g., baking, working [what kind of job?], running errands, volunteer work, taking care of children, visiting family/friends [list names], farm work)?* Greg would be at 4-H, school, or over at Robert's house. Gill would be fishing with older brother Bob, or helping with chores. Terry would be working, and I, Julie, when I was younger would be at choir practice or at Tina's house.

36. *Are their any life traumas the person remembers and still struggles with (e.g., death of a child or sibling, Holocaust, being abused)?* Her brother, Terrance, drowned in a river. My mom doesn't like water or the idea of us going swimming in rivers or lakes.

37. *What causes stress (e.g., noise, people, certain subject, getting dressed)?* When three or more people are talking. Very suspicious of people talking about her if she isn't included in the conversation. Doesn't like noise. Wants the kids to play outside.

38. *What calms them down (e.g., poetry, favorite song, massage, familiar activity, hug, bible verse)?* Listening to the birds chirp, the sound of raindrops, crossword puzzles. Sit next to her and say, "Your little brother Gill was your best friend." Looking at gardening magazines, getting her hair done, singing.

39. *Anything else that would bring this person joy?* Sneak her Bazooka bubblegum and Tootsie Pops (I will make sure she has her own stash to share with everyone). Bring her flowers. She loves when anyone shares their talent. Enjoys lotion on her feet and hands.

Tell her she is a "hard worker," or say, "You took such great care of Gill." Wink at her. Gossip with her.

40. *When you had a bad day, how did this person take care of you?* Listened to me, gave me a can of pop or made me chocolate chip cookies, encouraged me to take a nap or a walk, reassured me tomorrow will be different. If Mom was having a bad day, she would just say, "Get over it!"

41. *How did they put you to bed?* Gave us a bowl of cereal or ice cream. Sang to us "Sleep my child and peace attend thee," or just said, "Get to bed!"

42. *What would you put in a box to let everyone know who this person is?* Lotion, pictures of dad when he was young, her graduation picture, pictures of us kids when we were little, favorite CDs, gardening gloves, artificial pink rose or daisy, coffee mug, picture of her and Gill when they were young.

43. *How did they show you they loved you?* Listened, made me something to eat, touched my hand.

44. *What makes them feel loved?* Attention, being heard, sneak her sweets, tree hug, and a smile.

The sun will rise and set regardless. What we choose to do with the light while it's here is up to us. Journey wisely. —ALEXANDRA ELLE

Newfound Person

How Did They Love You?

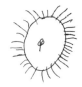

As professionals, we tend to say to families, "Your mom was agitated last night. What should we do?" Kids can't answer that question because we're focusing on Alzheimer's, and it's nearly impossible to figure out Alzheimer's. Instead, ask the children, "How did they take care of you? How did they love you when you weren't feeling well, when you had a bad day, or when you got hurt?" Kids can answer that. Consider…the way they cared for their children is how we can take care of them. Even if they can't communicate, if this is how they cared for their kids, it's familiar.

When you had a bad day, they…
- Hugged you (Bear hug or side hug?)
- Made you something to eat (Specifically what food?)
- Quoted a Bible verse (Which one specifically?)
- Went for ice cream (What's their favorite flavor?)
- Listened (It doesn't take words to make someone feel better.)
- Baked cookies (What kind?)
- Sang a silly song (Teach everyone the song.)

In my family, we punch each other on the shoulder and say, "Suck it up and deal with it. Stop being a baby!" In other words, it doesn't have to be butterflies and cupcakes. It just has to be familiar.

A young lady told me that when she visited her grandma, she would run inside the house and her grandma would reach down and touch her cheek, saying endearingly, "Oh, sweet girl." Now that her grandma is older, this young lady reaches over to her grandma's cheek and says, "Oh, sweet girl." Grandma has not forgotten this gesture of love.

When they put you to bed, they...

* Tucked you in (How many blankets? From high on your shoulders?)
* Said prayers (A specific prayer?)
* They just said, "GET TO BED!!!"

When they gave you a bath, they...

* Used bar soap (What brand?)
* Dried you with a warm towel (Warm theirs!)
* Added bubble bath (Or not.)
* Washed your hair in the bathtub (Or in the sink?)

My dad was always working when I was growing up and was physically abusive when he drank. Now he doesn't recognize me, but caregivers tell me he frequently asks for me, and when he is displeased he calls out my name. One afternoon I found him staring out the window with a very sad look on his face. "Hi, Dad. What's wrong?," I asked. He told me about his little girl, his daughter, and how much he missed her. "I don't think she loves me," he said. I asked my dad to tell me about her. What I heard was a tale about a father who did love his daughter but didn't know how to show it. He said, "I just wish I could tell her how much I love her." With tears in my eyes, I said, "She knows, Dad, she knows."

My mom verbally and physically abused us. Now she has Alzheimer's and I watch her give her caregivers hugs and joke with them. I don't understand.

If you were abused as a child, this alone gives you permission not to take care of them. You may not be able to see beyond the pain of your relationship to give the care they need.

Some parents have had difficulty showing their love to their own children. This moment may very well be the one that heals two people. Be open to the blessings of Alzheimer's.

My mother knows what buttons to push because she sewed them on. —A DAUGHTER

Newfound Forgiveness

Memory Box

What would you put in a box to let everyone know who your mom or wife is? Perfume, her favorite scarf, jewelry, a picture of her sister, love letters, lotion, recipe cards, a stethoscope because she is a nurse?

What would you put in a box to let everyone know who your dad or husband is? A specific tool he used; his cap, watch, cologne, tie; a newspaper? Don't forget one of the most important moments in a man's life. Nope, not his wedding day; yep, the purchase of his first vehicle. Resurrect a picture of him with his first vehicle. Far into dementia, they remember the make, model, year, color, and exactly how much they paid for it. But if you ask them, "When is your wife's birthday?" Hmmm…

When you move the person into someone else's care, it is imperative that you include this box. Then new caregivers and visitors can pick up the box and say, "Gary, is this your box? It has your name on it." Then they can go through the box together. Or the caregiver can get some work done, as Gary is occupied rummaging through his things. Please do not put any valuable items in this box because they will be gone tomorrow. Substitute things that resemble the real items.

A family shared how they filled a jar with memories, so moment after moment their mom could reach in the jar and pull out a memory.

Things to put in the jar: Pictures of a beloved pet; birdseed or a bird book; familiar lingo written on pieces of paper ("Our Sweet Pea"); children's drawings; a funny story; sweet treats; a picture of the home they lived in at the age they believe they are now; sheet music; song lyrics.

You can also get a jewelry box and untangle jewelry while you adorn her, embrace her hands, kiss her cheek, and bow to the "Queen."

Or consider…a music box, a hat box, a toolbox, a gardening box, a tackle box, a mystery box, a wedding box, or an empty box.

My mother is a hoarder and saves every empty box in the basement. She says, "You never know when you might need a box for birthday gift, Christmas gift, etc." I got one of those boxes and asked her, "What shall we put in this box?"
—JOEL KETCHER

The container you put it in won't always be a box. Jewelry goes in a jewelry box, tools belong in an old wooden toolbox, cooking utensils belong in a kitchen drawer, buttons in a tin. Do not use a plastic container because when you put a lid on it the person has no idea what is in there, and plastic isn't a familiar item.

We pulled out a very special box. The lace tablecloth was draped over the table by one of the ladies. The table was set by another lady, the crumpets served by another, and the tea poured by another. Sitting up straighter, pointing out pinkie fingers, they babbled and laughed about nothing but about everything.

I made Mom a memory box and the lights came on...for short moments. She identified a childhood friend and herself in a group picture! She smiled and just held onto some of the pictures. I also blew them up on my computer so they were big enough for her to see...and I can print as many copies as she wants.
—CHARLES

If someone doesn't have family, get an empty box and ask everyone to contribute something. During the holidays, go to thrift stores, garage sales, or your own closet to find things to fill a box, then wrap it up and give it as a gift. When things come up missing from the box, know that you created joy for others.

Smile: A curve that can set a lot of things straight. —UNKNOWN

Newfound Boxes

Life Reflection

Look around your home. Do you see pictures to remind you of special times? If someone who didn't know you looked at those pictures, they would just see people. You look at those pictures and you see a wonderful story behind each one.

Every person should have pictures around them that reflect their adventures in life. For the person with Alzheimer's, avoid using pictures from the recent past. Instead, pull out pictures from the age at which they are living in their mind. One exception to that rule is pictures of grandchildren. Everyone loves pictures of babies and kids. But the goal is to find old pictures of the person, including a picture of them around age eighteen, and pictures of a beloved grandparent, a childhood pet, their children (when they were young), and their wedding day.

Grandma would yank the fiftieth anniversary picture off the wall because Grandpa was having an affair with another woman. She didn't recognize her older self.

I suggest you keep the original pictures and have copies made to place in pretty picture frames. That way your precious photos won't get lost or be misplaced.

After making copies of treasured photos, write down the story for each (identifying the people in the photo) and place each story underneath its photo. Now anyone who enters their room can give them their memory back and get to know this person beyond the disease.

Avoid putting all the pictures in a photo album because they may not know where to find it if it is closed or put away. Sprinkle pictures everywhere for all to see!

I would do Dorothy's hair in the morning and within a few hours she would run her fingers continually through her hair until it stood straight up. Needless to say I was a bit frustrated because her hair always looked messy. One day her family brought in a picture of her when she was younger. Guess what her hairstyle was? Pulled straight back into a tight bun. I then understood that she was doing her hair instead of messing it up.

Pictures are like "old-timer's cash." They prompt memories of where this person has been and can provide entry points into their past.

They invite us to remember; that is, to take life apart, to look at it anew, and to put it back together again with joy, forgiveness, sorrow, and gratitude. Really, it allows us to close chapters of life with peace or to open them a crack just for a good laugh…or a good cry. —SISTER TERESA, S.P.

Newfound Picture

Music Does Wonders

Pull out old records and resurrect a record player. Simply seeing a record, with the needle perfectly placed, will set the tone for relaxation and contentment. You can also take the new (an iPod or smartphone), stroll over to the old (radio or record player), and pretend to turn it on while letting your iPod play. Play Big Band, Louis Armstrong, Glenn Miller, Guy Lombardo, Ella Fitzgerald, Bing Crosby, or Frank Sinatra. The list is beautiful and long.

Just seeing an old-style radio will trigger them to listen; many people sat around the radio every evening listening to popular radio shows like *The Lone Ranger, Roy Rogers, Gene Autry, Sky King, Tom Mix*, and *The Green Lantern*. What a treat that would be for all who are listening!

To add to the experience, shuffle through old record covers or pictures of radio show characters, like the Lone Ranger and Elvis Presley. When they see their face, or read the title, a moment in time is most likely to resurface. It's best to find a genre from their younger years, like the music they danced to on Friday nights or their favorite love song.

It's key is to have the record player, radio, or piano as the centerpiece in the main living room. If it is down the hall in another room, the person with dementia does not see it, and therefore it does not exist. With whatever you're playing, the most important thing is the quality of sound, so don't skimp on the cost. So, yes, get the expensive headphones that drown out all the background noise.

However, avoid playing music in the background while doing other things. For example, don't play music while trying to have a conversation, play a game, or eat dinner. They can only focus on one thing at a time, and music in the background is simply noise.

My church was well-known for having the best modern church music. I thoroughly enjoyed that music, but now suddenly I find I am distracted by

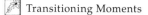

it. A few minutes of listening to the beat of the drums are enough to produce discomfort, even a headache.

Certain music can cause discomfort or be distracting. This person is your teacher, so find what music calms and relaxes them.

God did not leave me comfortless in my need for music to fill my soul. One day I was sorting through my record collection, and in that discard process that always comes at the end of a career or the end of life, I found an old George Beverly Shea record. It was one of the first so-called long play (33 rpm) records. Out of curiosity, I put it on my phonograph. From that old scratched record came Bev's deep voice singing simple old hymns. I sat back listening, then realized I was actually enjoying it. This music spoke to me. I eagerly played more of the old records with hymns. A sense of peace and enjoyment came over me as I listened to these records, which I had considered merely historical curiosities and put away years ago. And now I again have music to bless my soul.

—Excerpt from *My Journey into Alzheimer's Disease* by Robert Davis

Visiting a memory care community, a gentleman with his guitar in hand was singing old hymns. When he sang "Onward Christian Soldier," the people marched around the room. When he sang "I'll Fly Away," a gentleman waved his hat in the air with full enthusiasm, another person sang at the top of her lungs while clapping, and another closed her eyes in contentment. Though aged vocal cords and dementia hindered singing for some, many happy feet kept the beat. His "Jesus Loves Me" was sung and felt by all. This young man, with his deep, smooth voice, sang for an hour, and they wanted more.

Even if they can't communicate, sing their favorite song. They just might hit the pitch, sing every word, and not miss a beat. If you have a high soprano voice, lower your voice range. Please do not sing "Amazing Grace" in the high hymnal pitches, as research shows it is irritating. Absolutely sing "Amazing Grace" though, and don't be surprised when someone asks, "Who died?" People and events may be forgotten, but certain songs bring forth an array of feelings.

The lady who usually comes and goes because, "Mom is waiting for me at home," stayed in our circle today. When we began "Angels We Have Heard On High," her whole face lit up with a beautiful smile. When we got to the refrain "Glo-o-o-o-ria," she kept the smile, closed her eyes, and swayed gently. That's what it's all about: music of the heart and soul. —Sister Gloria, S.P.

Whenever a stressful moment arises, like a shift change, returning from your family reunion, or fatigue, simply sing in low tones a song with a steady beat. If you can't sing, just begin with the first three words and act like you can't remember: "What's that song? I'm looking over a four leaf clover...?" Familiar music lowers their blood pressure, slows down their heart rate, and changes their mood in a moment. Drums with a steady beat, nursery rhymes with a steady beat, or your calm voice with a steady beat: their heart rate will resonate with the beat.

One day at a memory care community, in my enthusiasm I belted out, "Rockin' Robin." People were shell-shocked. I guess we're not yet ready for rock 'n' roll, but I will try again because the baby boomers have arrived. —JOLENE

It might not yet be time for rock 'n' roll, but include drumming because a steady beat is innate in all of us. The first sound we felt and heard was our mother's heartbeat: a comforting, connecting sound—the rhythm of life. Research has shown that group drumming can reduce stress and inspire creativity and bonding, and it requires the use of both hemispheres of the brain. Drumming creates a joyful and meaningful experience without words: where memory fails, music speaks.

We were sitting in our drum circle. Sitting in a circle creates a sense of community and inclusion, and all are encouraged to share their own beats. I looked up and saw a gentleman gazing at the drums. He then began smiling and tapping out a rhythm on his knees. I asked him if he used to play the drums. There was no reply, but he continued smiling and tapping. The music started and so did the dancing of a few residents: a joyful connection. In this moment, we reconnected with our own unique inner rhythm.
—CYNDI BOOT, RHYTHMIC MEMORY: ENRICHING LIVES THROUGH DRUMMING

When Laurence Welk is on, I say, "Let's dance!" He says, "I'm not a good dancer," but we sway together. He likes the personal touch and making funny faces at me. Of course I give him a funny face back.
—A WIFE WHO LOVES HER HUSBAND

St. Augustine said, "Those who sing pray twice." So sing. Fill the space with music.

Take a deep breath and enjoy the rhythm of your day. —Cyndi Boot

Newfound Old Song

A Commercial about TV

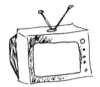

What's happening on TV is real for them. If someone gets shot on TV, then someone just got shot in front of them. If news of a hurricane or war pops up, they think it's happening right now even if it happened a month ago. When they experience hallucinations or confusion we blame it on Alzheimer's, when in reality they often are reacting to what they saw on TV.

My dad's dementia escalated to a whole new level when he was glued to the TV worried about the hurricane coming through.

When Donald Trump is on TV, he will hit the TV and say, "That son of a bitch. I wish he'd get out of here!"

On the flip side, if watching old westerns is a habit of a lifetime, then it will be calming. Curl up on the sofa and watch old musicals like *Oklahoma* or *The Sound of Music.* Choose upbeat content like the Shirley Temple movies, Lawrence Welk, shows featuring polka music, movies containing baby animals or babies, sports, or game shows such as *The Price is Right* (but you'd better have prizes in the mail). Even *I Love Lucy* has a story line too detailed to follow and is likely to lose their interest, but the humor may make you smile.

If they do like certain TV shows, videotape the shows without commercials so they can watch them over and over.

My mother called me and said she didn't know how she was going to feed all these people in her house. I went over to her house and no one was there, but the TV was on and she didn't know how to turn it off.

We were watching TV with my mom and out of the blue she said, "Girls put your knees together, they can see up your dress."

I noticed a lady in a wheelchair with a pained look on her face. I knelt in front of her and started singing "By the Light of the Silvery Moon." I didn't see a twinkle in her eye. Then I heard the roar of a TV in the adjacent room. The words were very harsh and seemed to be causing her pain. I slowly moved her into the dining room, where I said, "Let's sit in front of the window. It's such a lovely day." I commented on a little girl across the street and she replied, for the first time plainly and coherently, "Where's her mother?" I assured her that the little girl's mom was watching her out of the window. The look of pain vanished from her face.

Families tend to put TVs in the person's room because our generation cannot live without a TV. But their generation sat around a radio. Replace the TV with a CD player with radio so that they can (with assistance) enjoy *The Lone Ranger, Amos 'n' Andy,* or a baseball game. Would a man have behaviors if you put on his favorite baseball hat, turned on the game, and drank a cold beer with him? Absolutely not!

TV is not comforting unless it is familiar. Otherwise it's simply noise to them, which adds to their confusion. Good quality sound is helpful. Try using headphones to eliminate background noise. Or turn off the TV and simply enjoy the peace and quiet.

You and I have learned to tune out what we regard as background noise and background conversations…it is all "foreground" for her [his mom with Alzheimer's]. —DAVID DODSON GRAY

Newfound Entertainment

Ring, Ring, Ring

Telephones are a positive and a negative. When they see the phone, they're triggered to call you, not remembering that they called you five minutes ago. Now who is suffering? But…if the person is in a spin (see the chapter "The Spin"), sometimes the only way to get them out of it is to have someone give them a call.

> When my mother became upset and anxious, I would call one of her friends and have them call her. They would chitchat as they usually did. It changed my mom's mood instantly.

> My mom lives next door. When I visit her, she chats for a little while and then scoots me out the door. But when I call her on the phone, we have long talks as we always have.

If you want to continue chatting with this person, do not get them a cell phone because it will be nearly impossible for them to figure out something new.

> My mom calls: "Dear, I'm making an apple pie this morning. How many apples shall I peel?" Now, I wondered at this, as mom has always been an expert baker. "Well, Mother, I think six would be sufficient." A few minutes later the phone rings again: "This is your mother. I'm baking an apple pie and I am wondering how long should it be in the oven." I assured her of the approximate baking time. Forty-five minutes later: "Dear, this is your mother. Do you think it's time I take the apple pie out of the oven?" "Mother, it smells delicious." "Good, out it comes. I shall slice us each a piece, Dear." I live in Los Angeles and my mom lives in Indiana. We still have mother/daughter moments.
> —Gwendolyn de Geest

Trust me, you are going to miss your mother calling.

My mother calls me fifty times in the middle of the night worried that the furnace isn't working and the pipes might freeze. In the beginning, my husband would go over and reassure her by checking on the furnace. But now we just have an answering machine that tells my mom he will check on it in the morning.

When they are at home, you cannot stop a person from calling you fifty times. Consider the larger feeling…they are alone, or scared, or sad. This may be an indicator that it is time to have someone they trust come live with them or to move them into a care community, where someone is there 24/7.

You personally may want to get another phone line, but still keep the old number so they can call and hear your voice over an answering machine. When the phone becomes a problem (which it usually does), then have a young man in uniform tell them, "Your phone isn't working, Ma'am. Let me get it fixed for you." The phone never gets fixed. Or simply unplug it so it doesn't work.

It's a caregiver's role to intervene when someone wants to continually call family; have a number to call that has a busy signal or a number that will just ring and ring so they think no one is home, and assure the person you will try again later.

A lady wanted to call her husband, but he was no longer living. The caregiver called her own husband. As long as this lady heard a man's voice, she settled down.

A lady was looking for her dad, especially in the evening. Caregivers figured out that her dad was the one to tuck her in when she was a little girl. They made it part of her routine to call a male nurse working in another area and have him say, "Hi, Honey. I am working late tonight. I promise to tuck you in when I get home."

Two ladies were visiting in the backyard and there was a shovel stuck in the ground not far away. One lady sighed and said, "That's as far as he got spading for a garden…the worms looked so good he went fishing."

Newfound Ring

This Is Not Your Room!

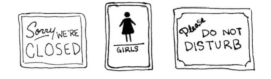

A major struggle with people with Alzheimer's is that they go in and out of other people's rooms. I'm going to give you some solutions.

There were a couple of gentlemen trying to get out through a locked door. A caregiver walked by and without missing a beat said, "Gentlemen, that is the ladies' bathroom." The men backed away from the door.

Find an artist to paint the doors at your dead-end hallways, or go online to order wallpaper with bookshelves and scenery to put on the doors. If you don't want this person to use the door then it cannot look like a door. That is the only solution. The easy answer is to paint the exit doors the same color as the wall. The door bar has to be painted too. In communities with elevators, do the same thing, and cover the buttons to match the wall.

Paint windows on the doors at the end of the hallways. Paint sceneries in rooms. Honestly, paint a beautiful view anywhere. Then add simple side curtains to create the illusion.

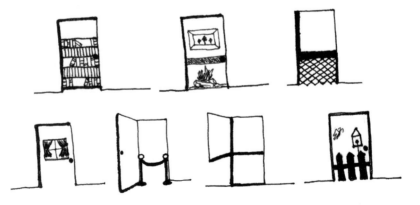

My sister-in-law is an artist, and I asked her to paint something beautiful in a memory care community I was helping to remodel. Her first layer of paint was of blue skies and soft clouds. One resident would come around the corner and say, "This is heaven, isn't it?" Then five minutes later he would come around the corner and again say, "This is heaven, isn't it?" She then added kittens, butterflies, a white picket fence, birds, and all sorts of flowers. Directly across from this wall, I created an indoor patio with rocking chairs and a mailbox. When people visited this memory care community they were questioning whether the people who lived here had Alzheimer's. It made me smile because I knew it was a success. They were functioning better because the environment supported the disease, and the person. —Jolene

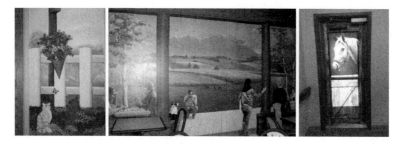

If you are still caring for the person at home and you don't want them to use the door, simply put a lock at the top of the door. The person won't look up or figure out a new lock. The locks can also be put on the outside of the doors so the person is secure inside the house. Another trick is to place a black rug or mat in front of the door. To them it is a black hole they won't step over.

The person only knows what they see right now, and if what they see doesn't look familiar (which it doesn't), then they will want to find the nearest door to find a place that is familiar. The only solution is to camouflage or hide the exit door around the corner. Dead-end hallways literally are dead-end problems.

Close some doors today not because of pride, incapacity, or arrogance, but simply because they lead you nowhere. —Unknown

---

Newfound Hidden Door

It's Saturday Night!

When they were growing up they took baths, not showers. Take the word *shower* out of your vocabulary. What did they call it? Spit bath, sponge bath, washed up, cleaned up, PTA? Have you heard of the PTA? Pits, Tits, and Ass. Yes! Whatever their lingo, use it!

As we age we lose our sense of smell, so, no, they cannot tell they need to get washed up. If you approach with, "It's time for your bath," they will simply reply, "I just took one this morning," but really it's been a week or maybe a month. Instead, what would get this person up out of their chair: dinner, getting the newspaper, the Pledge of Allegiance? Whatever it is, once they're up, walk toward the bathroom, and when you get near the door say, "Let's get washed up for [insert reason]." Now what would this person would get washed up for? "It's Saturday night. Church is tomorrow. You get the first hot tub." "There's a business meeting today. Let's get cleaned up." "Company is coming. Let's freshen up." "Harold is coming. I promise to make you look beautiful."

> *A clever nutty caregiver would put a little toothpaste or syrup in her hand, walk up to the person, pat them on the knee, and say, "Well hello, Sunshine! (Pause…) What's this on your knee?" Then the person would touch their knee, feeling the stickiness. (Why the knee: because they can see and feel it there.) Then she would whisper, "I have some other pants. Let's go change."*

Reasons bathing causes fear

Noises alone can cause fear (fan, water running, people talking). They get colder than cold: warm towels, warm robe, 102 degrees in the room…and they are freezing. Past fears are triggered: drowning, being molested. No matter the reason for their fear, the point is, stop blaming their reaction on the disease. When we blame it on Alzheimer's, we are forgetting one valuable question. *Why?* Why are they reacting like this?

Habits of a lifetime

How did they get washed up at the age at which they are living in their mind? Did they typically wash up in the morning or in the evening? How much water did they use? Probably very little: truly a spit bath in a small basin with a washcloth and Lava soap. Did they wash their hair in the sink? If so, shampooing their hair in the shower with water running over their eyes is unfamiliar. Were they an extremely private person who might have dressed in the closet? Respect their privacy: turn your head and hand them the towel. Reassure them: "I won't look."

If you are their child, how did they give you a bath? This is how we can get them washed up, too. ☺

Environment

Walk into the bathing room. What do you see? What do you feel?

* *Cold:* Radiating panel and warming closet so everything is warm.
* *White tiles, white floors:* Feels institutional and cold. Warm red hues make us feel warmer.
* *Too big, no privacy:* Install pretty curtains to create smaller spaces.
* *Crowded; has become a place for storage:* Clutter creates confusion. They will wonder, "What are they going to do to me in here?"
* *Lighting:* Increase the light level so they don't feel like they are in a darkened room, and add a dimmer switch to suit different tastes.
* *Mid-range color towels:* Place them on the shower seat so they can see where they are sitting and are no longer cold.
* *Mirrors:* Remove or cover up the mirrors with a window shade, or slap wet paper towels on the mirror to break up the reflection. A person with dementia perceives the mirror as a window and will think that someone is peeking.
* *Bathing visuals:* Place bathing items directly in their line of vision—pictures of children in the bathtub, a rubber ducky, a pretty towel—so they see that this is where we get washed up.
* *Belts, Depends, chrome on tub:* Anything clinical, put in a cupboard or cover with a robe or muumuu.
* *Bidet:* Yes, please! Install a bidet to clean private areas. This is much less intrusive than using your hand.
* *Barber or salon chair:* Yes, please! And with a sink so they can have a familiar experience.

Preserving modesty

When getting them undressed, pretend: "Whoops, I didn't mean to spill that," or "I'm just going to wash your feet." Then remove one piece of clothing at a time.

* Sew two towels at the top corners to create a "poncho" to put over the person, or cover their lap with a towel. When the towels are wet, use them to clean the person. Have a dry poncho ready to put on after the shower/bath to dry them.
* Cut a hole in the middle of an old sheet and use it to cover the person completely while bathing. Wash one area at a time and then cover it.
* Don't hover over them. Do something else: clean, read a book, or pretend you are looking for something (quietly).
* Three bathrobes: one to begin, one to wash in, and a warm one to have ready when they are finished "washing up."

Bathing tidbits

* Start the bathing process by washing the safest, least intimidating areas (feet, arms).
* Avoid shower heads. Their skin is very sensitive and the shower's spray may cause pain or fear. If you must use a shower head, at least cover it with a washcloth.
* If the person is still mobile, use a shower seat in the bathtub because it is more familiar.
* Fill the tub one-third full before the person is in the room to cut back on noise.
* Use bubbles and play an old-style radio with soothing music.
* To provide the person with the illusion of control, hand them their own "stuff": washcloth, soap, cup (not the shower head ☺).
* Sponge bath or "spit bath": Fill the sink with water and give the person a washcloth and a bar of soap (liquid soap is unfamiliar).
* One task at a time. *Don't rush!!!*
* When washing their hair, hold a washcloth against their forehead so water doesn't get in their eyes. (Better yet, have the person hold the washcloth.)
* Have a man hold a warm washcloth over his face and lean back. This is a familiar position from when he got a shave at the barber. It's also less threatening because he can't see what you're doing.
* Focus all your attention on this person.

* Use a gentle touch, and pat dry rather than rub. Their skin is paper thin and very sensitive.
* Use soft towels. How many towels? Depends on the person. One lady thinks she has to do the laundry, so one small towel. Another person is concerned about privacy, so twelve towels.
* Magic words: "I am here if you need me." "I understand. We will take it slowly." "I will be careful." "Can I help ...?"
* Bribe them: "After this, we will get a big bowl of ice cream." Provide whiskey (apple juice warmed up) before, during, and after the bath.
* With businessmen make an appointment and have him sign his name.
* Check water temperature on the inside of your wrist. Remember that what is warm to you may be hot to them.
* Stick to a routine.
* Kick-start: Begin by putting your hand over their hand and start washing their face, then let go.
* Say "Please ...," "May I ...?," and "Thank you."
* If you are comfortable giving a bath, they are more likely to be comfortable with you.
* Say: "I'm sorry. I didn't mean to hurt you." "I'm sorry. That was my fault."
* Include the person: "I will wash this arm, you wash your other arm."
* Act naive: "I don't know how to give a bath. Will you show me?" (Provides the illusion of control.)
* Distract them by talking about a favorite subject (e.g., fishing, cooking).
* Tell her, "You are going to be queen for a day!"
* Sing with them. Sing for them.
* Use yes/no questions: "Would you like ...?"
* Make spa coupons that say, "This is a special treat from your kids."
* Have them bathe a babydoll while you are bathing them.
* Play Good Guy/Bad Guy: Bad Guy begins the bath, and when the person becomes upset, Good Guy comes in and says, "Get out of here! That's not okay! I'm sorry, June. She should not have done that. May I help you get washed up?" They are more likely to cooperate with Good Guy, who saved day.

George didn't want to take a shower, and it had been two weeks. A caregiver called George on the phone and acted like his wife. She told him they were going to visit friends that night, and he'd better get cleaned up. It worked!

Someone asked me what my magic is with the lady who is difficult to get washed up. My answer: "I show her kindness every day. She trusts me."

—Jerry Ritari

A lady resisted taking a bath so the caregiver put on an apron. "I bet her mom wore an apron. Women in aprons are warm, loving moms and grandmas."

Our home has a scale in the tub and we say that the doctor needs their weight. We also get our male caregivers to put on a white jacket, becoming the doctor who recommends a hot bath for therapy.   —A bathing expert

Avoid using whirlpool tubs with bubbles because these bubbles look like boiling water. The best tub I have researched and caregivers really like is the Parker Bath from ArjoHuntleigh, Inc. It looks like a tub, has little chrome, fills up ahead of time so there is no waiting, and slowly leans back so the water goes under the person.

As they were lowering Therstin into a tub, he yelled, "Pig! Pig!" He was a farmer and thought they were lowering him into boiling water. This is how farmers get the skin off pigs.

A lady stated with much resistance, "I don't want soup! I don't want soup!" To her the Jacuzzi was a pot of boiling soup.

Consider that they are getting partially cleaned up throughout the week: their hair gets washed at the beauty salon, and we clean their private areas if they are incontinent. All we have left are the legs, torso, and arms, which may easily be cleaned with a traditional sponge bath.

The best solution when anyone is struggling is to go back to "bed baths": they are safely in their room, in their bed, covered up with a heavy blanket. Start with the least intimidating areas and work your way down. Roll the person onto their side to get their back and finish with lotion (that you have warmed up in a basin of hot water). Hand them a hot wet washcloth to wash their own private area, if possible. Use no-rinse soap and dry shampoo. I guarantee if you go back to bed baths you will not have all the behaviors (better called *reactions*) you are having with showers. This person cannot change the fear that comes up. We are the only ones who can change how we get them washed up.

You don't have to submerge someone to get them clean. Respect the person's right to say no. No one has ever died because they didn't get a bath!!! If they resist, leave and try again later.

A nutty caregiver in her seventies who as been a caregiving her entire life shares her wisdom: "I promise them back rubs, sing, try to keep them warm, and reassure that l will get it done quickly. Or I will say, 'You're being really brave because this is difficult.' If they scream, let them, and reassure them, 'I know this is hard. It's almost over. You're being so brave!' I am a 159-year-old grandma. I can spoil them, kiss them on their cheek, and get them to behave."

There are caregivers who simply have a gift. Smart communities will recognize this gift, bestow the title of Bathing Expert or Bath Whisperer, and pay this person more for their expertise. If a caregiver gives a bath on Wednesday, then a different caregiver gives a bath on Friday, how does that make the person feel? Vulnerable, confused, and wondering, "What is this person doing?" But when it's the same face and the same routine…you get into a rhythm. If you have found a Bath Whisperer, count your many blessings.

A friend of mine was the only one able to get this lady washed up. She said, "I really like this lady, and others don't because she can be difficult. But I say to her, 'June, if you let me help you, I promise to make you beautiful.' And I do make her beautiful by combing her hair and putting on her favorite dress. It's quite simple."

To finish up: give them a back rub, gently comb their hair, apply lipstick, put on his cologne to "wow the women," and of course tell them how beautiful or how handsome they look.

I inquired, "Sister Charles, how do you get such beautiful skin?" She smiled and touched her cheek. "You rub it with Love everyone once in a while." —Love to Sisters of Providence

---

Newfound PTA

Where's the Outhouse?

One of the main reasons people with dementia are incontinent is that they cannot find the bathroom. When the person wakes up in the middle of the night they see two doors: one with a light under it and another that is dark. Choosing the one with the light, they walk into the hallway where there are lots of doors. Where's the bathroom? They check each door until they cannot hold it any longer.

Or, the person walks out the door, turns right, and pees. He is peeing over the back patio as he always has. His body will remember the motion it has been doing for a lifetime.

What color is the toilet? *White.* What color are the bathroom walls? *White.* What color is the floor? *Off white.* They can't see white on white. If they can't see it, they can't use it. Do you know what I learned while earning my interior design degree? Colored paint doesn't cost more than white paint. Paint the wall behind the toilet a midrange color so they see the toilet.

What color is the shower seat? *White.* What color is the shower stall? *White.* Placing a midrange-colored towel on the shower seat would help them to see it. But what color are the towels? *White.* Hmmm…do you see a pattern here?

Suggested changes
* Leave the bathroom door open with light on after they fall asleep. If they see the toilet they are more likely to use it.
* Replace the bathroom door with a shower curtain.
* NO POCKET DOORS!
* Replace the toilet seat with a different color.
* Paint the wall behind the toilet a midrange color.
* Paint a half moon (outhouse symbol) on the door.

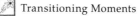

* Paint the bathroom door a different color from the other doors: "It's the blue door over there." They keep the ability to distinguish colors far into the disease.
* Remove the mirror if they don't recognize their reflection; they won't use the bathroom because "someone is already in there."
* Place the toilet paper in direct sight.
* Have storage cabinets in the bathroom so everything is accessible to clean up accidents.

What are the nonverbal cues when someone has to pee? Leaning to one side, pacing, restlessness, squirming, holding privates, fidgeting with pants, getting up to leave...Make note of these cues.

Don't ask, "Do you need to use the bathroom?" The answer will be "No." Instead, make a statement: "Time to get washed up for dinner." Then when you are in the bathroom, simply say, "Better use the john before we go." What did they call the bathroom in their younger years? Privy, two-holer, john, outhouse, latrine, lavatory, powder room, chamber pot? Use their lingo and place a sign on the door as a way-finding clue. A picture of a toilet on the door is not a way-finding clue.

How did they say I have to go to the bathroom?

"I gotta see a man about a horse."
"I have to shake the rattlesnake."
"I gotta see Mrs. Jones."
"I gotta drain my brain."
"I gotta feed the chickens."
"I gotta shake the dewdrops off the lily pad."
"I gotta take a leak."
"I gotta pee."
"I gotta take a piss"
"I gotta take a shit!"

Oh, he shouldn't talk that way! Do you want this guy continent or incontinent? Then you'd better learn to say, "Tom, is it time to take a shit?"

It could be as discreet as, "I need to take a walk." Or they may only remember how to say *bathroom* in their native language.

A lady pushed on the door that goes outside: "Let me out! Let me out!" She was labeled an "elopement risk." Someone eventually figured out that when she did this, she actually needed to use the outhouse.

Fixing leaks

I have been asked how to deter men from urinating in wastepaper baskets, wall heaters, closets, fake trees, and other areas. I think it's funny when we think we are going to get men to *use* the bathroom. At what age did they learn they can pee anywhere they want to? Three years old. You think you are going to change them?

The wastepaper basket looks like a hole and the wall heater a urinal. The fake tree, of course, is a real one. So I say, more trees! At least they hit something! That tree is cheaper to replace than the carpet. Smart memory care communities have "potty plants." They fill big pots with kitty litter, add a fake plant, and place them at end of hallways. It works. Change your mind and start placing wastepaper baskets everywhere. Install wall heaters up high or put plastic covers over them.

Girlie posters, girlie posters, girlie posters. If you want men to use the bathroom, you need to give them a reason to go in there. Not the girlie posters of today, but from their generation.

A lady who had grown weary of cleaning up after accidents knew that a man liked Marilyn Monroe. So, she placed Marilyn Monroe pictures in the places where she didn't want him to urinate. She said it worked…but I forgot to ask her where he's peeing now. (Isn't this fun?!?)

You could also hang three pictures across from the toilet, one below the other: a picture of his motorcycle, a picture of his farm, and a picture of his favorite movie star. He goes into the bathroom and looks at the top picture, placed at eye level, then you point to the picture below that, then to the bottom picture. Now he is almost in squatting position, and you lean him back. Then, hand him *Hustler* or *Reader's Digest*. Don't forget to turn on the water. Or just take him outside to pee. The question to answer is: Where did they pee at the age at which they are living in their mind? (Cornfield?) As the disease progresses some women will squat again.

My husband has always peed on our back fence, so I took part of the back fence to the memory care community and put it in his shower with green turf on the floor. He is still peeing on the back fence.

What color is the toilet? What color is the water? This man cannot see where to point. Make the toilet water blue, or get red fingernail polish and paint a bullseye at the bottom of the toilet, or throw in some Fruit Loops. Who knows what will work?

To unbuckle their pants, ask the person to place their hands on your shoulders and ask if they would help hold you up: "Thank you for holding me up. You are strong." Or it may be less intrusive if you stand behind them when unbuckling their pants. Depends on the person.

Practice being quiet and invisible by placing yourself to the side of or behind the person. Placing your hand lightly on their shoulder may stop them from getting up and down. Another person may feel more comfortable if you hold their hand and chat a lot of nonsense…and laugh with them.

Some days, when "accidents" happen, I have to clean her up, of course. And I can tell she's not very happy with the world at all as she says, "What the hell are you doing?" I reply, "Getting you dressed, Sweetie." When I'm finished I say, "There, all pulled up and you're cozy warm. Okay." I know that when the cleaning up is over and she's clean (and lovely again), she's forgotten the bad stuff and she'll hold me close and just say, "I love you, Honey." We just feel very close and stand there together for a few moments, calm and happy. The shortness of memory that Alzheimer's brings is, of course, often a godsend. Most of the time BMs go into the toilet, and that's a moment of joy for me. My wife is not even aware that she's had a BM. But I make a big celebration of it and do a little jig in front of her. So we have a laugh, despite her probably thinking that I'm a crazy person! That's the type of moment of joy that is mutual! —ALAN ROSS, HUSBAND AND CAREGIVER*

Incontinence is the number one reason husbands move their wives into a care community. Men have not been trained to clean up messes, but there also seems to be so much shame around it. Families are ashamed when they discover the person is putting dirty underwear in the back of drawers and other creative spots to hide their accident. The person throws the underwear away, and the family can't figure out why the kitchen towels and washcloths are missing. The person is trying to fix the problem without anyone knowing. Rightfully so, because in their generation when they wet their pants or wet the bed, they got in trouble. Make it no big deal: "Underwear is cheap. I will pick up some more."

A daughter took me to her mom's bathroom where there were at least twenty boxes of Kotex pads.

Well, Mom was a little incontinent and didn't want anyone to know, and she was paranoid she would not have her "safety blanket." Sometimes she even got confused and bought tampons.

If the person is incontinent during the day, whisper, "You must have sat in a little water. Let's change so you feel better." Make it no big deal and it becomes no big deal.

A lady would pinch the female caregivers while toileting her, but if a male caregiver came in, she was sweet as pie. I took a black marker, made a mustache out of paper, and taped it under my nose. She never pinched me again. —WENDA K. GODFREY

To affect the quality of the day, that is the highest of arts. —HENRY DAVID THOREAU

Newfound Outhouse

Suppertime!!!!!

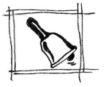

When I was a kid and the meal was ready, I would yell, "Suppertime!!!" My job was to set the table with my little brother. What are your traditions? Blessing the food? Dad sitting at the head of the table? Mom wearing an apron? Now incorporate these during the meals: "Would you help me set the table?" One at a time hand them place mats, then glasses, then napkins. However they help you, say, "Thank you for all your help. Go relax. Dinner will be ready in ten minutes."

What did their dining room look like? A buffet filled with china? Portraits of food? Spoon rack? Wallpaper? If you have a large room, break it up into smaller spaces. White light is best for the aging eye; however, be sure the intensity of the light can be adjusted by adding a dimmer switch. Reducing visual distractions and noise may be one of the most powerful changes you can make.

When setting the table, differentiate layers: solid-colored place mat, different-colored plate, and a different-colored napkin. Invite the person to the meal and talk about food on the way: "Join us for dinner. We are having..." Being invited to eat is important, and so is structured seating: "Joe, would you like to sit by Fred?" "Sara, would you like to sit by the window?" Hand the person a hot wet washcloth to "wash up."

There was a lady who would not eat in the dining room. We discovered that she was a farmer's wife, and her tradition was to feed the men, and then she would eat in the kitchen later.

Before meals have them help prepare the food by tearing lettuce, snapping beans, buttering bread, shucking corn, peeling potatoes, or pouring beverages. It's helpful for them to nibble on sweet or salty foods to increase saliva before the meal is served.

When my daughter turned two, she didn't need a sippy cup anymore. What did she do when I gave her a glass of milk? Poured it all over her food. I thought of Thirsten: Every meal he would pour his milk over his food. I corrected him every day, but did he change? No. I wish I would've given him a sippy cup or a glass with a lid and straw. Some will question whether that's age appropriate, but the better question is, does it work? Or better yet, is pouring milk on his food hurting him? No. Let it go.

As the disease progresses, their developmental level regresses. What is this person's developmental level?

What if you gave a one-year-old child a plate of food, salt and pepper shakers, two glasses, and three utensils? They would play. If the person is "playing," offer one item at a time.

Do kids come to the table, sit down, and not get up throughout the whole meal? No. Allow people with dementia to nibble "on the go."

Do kids eat when they are not hungry? No. Loss of appetite (and thirst) is a normal part of aging. It doesn't mean there's something wrong.

Do kids eat food they don't like? No. Serve foods they like and make all other food resemble it. Everything looks like a pie...quiche!

A gentleman had a stroke and wasn't eating. His wife brought him two pieces of fried chicken and he ate it! The next day she brought him four pieces and he ate it all!

A lady loved ice cream cones so her food was mashed up and put in a cone. Potatoes were vanilla ice cream and carrots were sherbet, and she ate on the go.

Ron will ask, "Do I like that? I just like the old things. I don't like the new things." He will only eat familiar foods. —A WIFE

How would your kids feel if they didn't have any snacks to nibble on? CRABBY. When we nibble, we relax. Have goodies available day and night. Have a pot of soup on the counter, little bags of chips, and snack jars 24/7 for caregivers, families, and the person who wakes up in the middle of the night.

What finger foods do kids like? Prior to serving, cut up everything into finger foods. Cheese slices, sandwiches (cut into four squares, without the crust), saltine crackers, graham crackers, smoothies, yogurt, Jell-O Jigglers, dry cereal, raisins, hot dogs (sliced along the way), little

muffins (big ones are messy), toast with peanut butter and jam or cinnamon and sugar, pancakes (rolled up with sugar), grapes, carrot/
broccoli/cauliflower sticks (boil to soften), cold green beans from a can
(yes, my kids and I love those), cherry tomatoes, strawberries, cookies,
ice cream…and the list goes on and on. Anything can be made into
a sandwich. Let go of silverware by wrapping food up in tortillas
or lettuce.

*I had a family very upset because Mom was eating her salad with her fingers.
But she was eating her salad! When we tried to help her she didn't eat because
she wanted to be independent!* —NATALIE

Older people are overwhelmed when they see large food portions
because they have been taught to clean their plates. Use a saucer-size
plate with teaspoon-size portions. If food has already been served, take
one-quarter of each serving and cover the rest up with a napkin. If they
don't see it, it doesn't exist. Increase nutrient density, not portion size,
by putting food into muffin tins and freezing them.

*Alice, a petite lady, would bang her walker on the table and walk away. She
couldn't eat that much food. When we served her food on a smaller plate, with
teaspoon-size portions, she ate her whole meal.*

If a person has disruptive or distasteful eating habits, have them sit
in a place visually away from the majority of people.

*I was asked for suggestions on how to stop a lady from yelling, a gentleman
from getting "up, down, up, down, up down," and another from pulling out
her dentures during mealtimes. There were approximately twenty-five people
eating at the same time in a large space. Trays were clanging, music was on
in the background, and staff was walking around. I knew right away it was
the environment triggering the "behaviors." I asked them to show me other
places available for dining. We came upon a wonderful small room that had
a kitchenette and simple table. They told me this was reserved for families
to visit and eat. My question: "Do the families live here?" The first priority
should always be the people who live here. People who have difficulty during
mealtimes are now eating better here.*

Create a social atmosphere by eating with them. Turn off the TV,
put on an apron, and start a conversation. That doesn't include talking
about what happened over the weekend with your co-worker.

Bring the person to the table only when the food is ready, and allow ample time to eat. No rushing! If the person is in a wheelchair, be sure they are at a proper height for the table. Help the person to "sit up straight" (elbows above the table), and ask their permission before you push them in.

There are many reasons they may not be eating: You haven't sat down yet. Too much noise! (The number one reason!) The person cannot start the motion (place your hand over their hand and assist with two bites). Their dentures may be uncomfortable or the food is too hard. They may have pain. They don't like the metallic taste of food (a side effect of medication; dispense medications before or after meals—NOT DURING!).

If they are unable to see directly in front of them, figure out where they can see by placing their favorite food in a colored bowl. Most plates are white and therefore white foods (potatoes, eggs, noodles) can't be seen. Try putting gravy or syrup over everything, and serve eggs sunny side up. Or serve on a different-colored plate (e.g., Fiesta dinnerware).

Avoid having too many choices. Offer one item at a time, in separate bowls, and wait until they are finished before you give them the next item.

My little boy and I were visiting a memory care home. Staff saw this as an opportunity to invite a lady who wouldn't come out of her room to eat with us. She was eating her bowl of salad, doing just fine, when a staff person came over and moved her unfinished salad to the side. Then they set down a plate of food. Next thing I know, she dumped her salad onto her plate, stuck her fork in it, and left the table. Let them finish!!!

When we serve juice, jelly, and butter in a sealed container, they lose their independence because they have to ask someone to open it. Better to put butter on a butter dish, jelly in a jelly jar. When we put cereal in a plastic container, they don't know what is in there so they won't utilize it independently.

A lady was known as a "feeder," but when a box of cornflakes was left on the table, she came over and poured herself a bowl. Seeing the box triggered her.

* Use wide-rim soup bowls or cereal bowls with straight sides to ease scooping. Serve soup in a coffee cup; drinking is easier than using a spoon.

* What did they eat and how did they eat? From a black lunch box? A brown paper bag? Alone, or with others? At a certain restaurant? (Put meals in a bag from that restaurant.)
* Did they prefer picnics? Add a red and white checkered tablecloth.
* Give them oranges and bananas because they are a treat for this generation and it's exercise to peel them.
* Say "it's time for coffee," not "snack time."
* Popcorn poppers and bread makers are amazing for "smells."

Assisted dining (not feeders)

* It's important not to over help.
* Sit in front of them, not to the side, because of failing peripherals.
* Tell the person what you are giving them.
* SLOW DOWN!
* Talk in a soothing voice and don't talk to others over the person.
* To trigger swallowing, start with ice cream or rub their throat.
* Allow them to swallow completely before giving them another bite.
* Place a spoon on their lower lip and leave it there until they take it.
* Prunes taste better warmed up.

Before and after meals, pass around warm wipes/washcloths to "wash up." After meals ask for their help to move chairs, pick up plates, or wipe off tables. Those who aren't mobile can wipe down place mats.

When someone wants to pay for the food and they don't have any money, here are two possible answers: "You have worked hard all your life. This is Uncle Sam's way of paying you back." Or, "This one is on me. You get the next one." Or let them write out a fake check.

In the early stages, they will eat more than they usually do because they forgot they just ate. Serve smaller meals more often. To extend the mealtime, involve the person in the preparation: toast bread, spread the mayo, cut tomatoes, wash lettuce (again and again), slice meat, then let the person know, "It's still in the oven."

Reduce their carb intake by having healthy foods front and center. Place the "sweets" in the cabinet behind a curtain. When they open the door, they won't see the sweets, but you know where they are. Get long-lasting treats like popcorn, gum, and lollipops.

Families who are concerned about weight gain, let it go! People with Alzheimer's passing away because of being overweight is unheard of. Let them eat while they will eat.

So long as you have food in your mouth you have solved all the problems for the time being. —Franz Kafka

Newfound Treat

Get Your Zzz's

Fatigue is a major cause of behaviors in all people, period, whether or not they have dementia. Naps, naps, naps!

A gentleman who was not able to sleep became disoriented, incoherent, and lethargic. Caregivers warmed up a towel and put a sock filled with rice into the microwave, then placed the towel over his head, put the sock over his shoulders, and sat with him. He finally fell asleep. The next day he was a different man. He joined in the discussion, laughed, and made jokes. It was a night-and-day difference when he got his much needed rest.

A gentleman would be put to bed, only to be up wandering around again. Staff asked his wife what his "habits" were when sleeping. She said he never wore pajamas; he slept in the nude. Staff had been putting pajama clothes on him, which to him meant that it was time to get up and start the day.

Any older person, whether or not they have dementia, should be allowed to wake up on their own time. What if you woke up a child in the morning before it was time? Or your child didn't get a nap today? Not a pretty sight! It's the same for someone with dementia.

We all have different needs. Some of us are night owls and some of us are morning people. Whatever the case, you are fighting a losing battle if you're trying to change someone's timetable.

When I get there, I'll be up all night and people will be all over me trying to get me to bed. You'll find me sleeping on a couch or maybe even in a chair. Don't assume I will sleep in a bed, and don't put me to bed early because it's easier for you. —Linda

It's also their right to stay up as late as they want. So many times we fight with the person to get them to go to bed. I wonder, who are we really trying to serve? The person or us? It makes it much easier on us when they are safely tucked in, sleeping the night away. If you're waking people up every two hours to check on them…Stop!!! That is insane!

The trouble with being on your feet all day, walking from one end of the building to the other, is that your legs get tired as well as the rest of your body. Caregivers know that. Add to that the fact that you're ninety, and you would really get tired.

It was time for Sara's nap. We aides took turns walking Sara to her room, helped her get her feet on the bed, covered her up, and left the room. A few feet down the hall, we'd hear the shuffle of her short, choppy steps. We looked back and there was Sara, gaining on us. The time we spent trying to get her to lie down was wasted.

"You need to lie down for a nap. Aren't you tired, Sara?" "Yes," she admitted. "Well, why won't you stay in bed then and take a nap?," I asked. "Because I want you to stay here with me." Sara's plaintive voice held an unspoken plea.

There we had it. She was lonely and fearful of being left in that empty room. She was in a large place where the sounds of doors banging, a variety of voices, and loud alarms seemed endless. In her confusion, she feared everything around her and what she heard. Now I understood why she kept following us out of the room.

I pulled up a chair, sat down by her bed, held her hand, and promised I would stay with her. Fighting sleep for a few minutes, Sara peeked over at me from slit eyelids to make sure I was still there. Her hand finally went limp in mine, and she breathed deeply in a sound sleep. Then I slipped out of the room.

Sitting by her bedside to give her peace of mind took far less time than walking her back to her room repeatedly. —FAY RISNER

The key is to leave someone with a peaceful feeling before they fall asleep. Lying down with someone for a few minutes is quite possibly all they need. (Look out…you may fall asleep yourself.)

A wonderful CNA shared this story. "When I put a lady to bed, I reassured her, 'The chickens are fed, the kids are in bed, and I stoked the fire. You get your rest.' When I said this to her, she slept through the night. But when I didn't reassure her, she was incontinent every two hours. Our goal is to make them feel like everything is okay before they nod off."

Suggestions to help them get their zzz's

* Expose them to sunlight. There are "light boxes" that mimic outdoor light to provide more Vitamin D. This will help lift their mood and help them sleep better.
* Keep people physically active during the day. (See the "Walking, Walking, Walking" chapter.)
* Establish a calming evening routine.
* Find foods to eat that promote better sleep.
* Eliminate stimulating activities after 7:00 p.m.
* Put on an extra blanket an hour after the person has fallen asleep to keep them warm.
* If the person is used to sleeping with someone else, get a body pillow and spray it with the cologne or perfume of the other person.
* Read poetry or rhymes, or sing quiet songs; a steady beat or rhythm is like a lullaby.
* Use white noise. It's a little machine that makes a subtle noise that is soothing to fall asleep to. (What was their childhood evening noise?)
* Fulfill habits of a lifetime: sleeping with a feather pillow, sleeping with the fan on, sleeping with a night-light, ensuring the room is pitch dark, etc.
* Allow the person to sleep in their own bed, no matter where they move.
* Ask if they have to use the bathroom before lying down.

A lady would not calm down. She paced up and down the hall. The hairdresser just so happened to stop by and didn't understand. This same lady was always relaxed when getting her hair done. So she walked the lady into her beauty shop and set her under the hair dryer. The only comment made was, "And the world goes away." Then she nodded off. What's in her room today? An old-style hair dryer.

My grandma would fight getting undressed for bed at night because she was convinced someone was going to steal her left shoe. (We still haven't figured out why it was only her left shoe.) My mom stepped in and requested that they let her keep her shoes on until she fell asleep. The battle was resolved. Choose your battles wisely. —Renae Smothers

How did your parents put you to bed? Because quite possibly how they put you to bed is how you can put them to bed.

My daughter shared with me that when her little boy was a baby, he would have crying fits that seemed to have no discernible cause. To soothe him, she would wrap him in a blanket and then place her arms around him, holding him gently along his sides.

I decided to try this with a resident at work who frequently becomes anxious and tearful and complains of pain. I had her cross her arms over her chest, hugging herself, and then I tucked a soft blanket around her. Next, I sat on a stool in front of her, placing my arms along the sides of her thighs. We didn't talk; we just sat quietly. She began to visibly relax and was then able to fall asleep. —GRETCHEN MELLBERG

I met a lady who had been working night shifts since she was seventeen, and now she was seventy-seven. I thought I'd better ask: "What do you do when they wake up in the middle of the night?" She said, "First, I ask if they have to use the bathroom. Then I take hold of their hand and say, "Get your rest, Dear. I promise it will be better in the morning." It's not so much her words but her tone of voice and touch that leave a secure feeling.

They also only know what they see right now. When they wake up in the middle of the night and see this lady with gray hair and an apron, who do they see? Grandma. Who do with feel safe with? Grandma.

Now, I would like you to imagine a man working the night shift. Nice guy, but when he walks into the room, what is she thinking? Intruder!!! If a man wants to work the night shift he needs to wear a gray wig with an apron or be handsome enough to invite to bed. ☺

While they are still at home and you're not able to sleep because the person is "up, down, up, down," medication is an option. But a glass of wine or shot of whiskey may be the best medication. Sleep is vital for both of you!!!

People who can fall asleep quickly freak me out…
I mean, don't they have thoughts? —MINIONS

Newfound Zzz's

Enhanced Moments

Touch many…radiate your warmth. —JOLENE

So You Wanna Visit?

U nderstand that people with Alzheimer's may not recognize you. There's no need to put it to the test by saying this very common phrase: "My name is Helen. Do you remember me?" If you sense they are wondering who you are, simply introduce yourself by your first name and visit as a friend or a stranger.

"Hi. What a long day! Would you mind if I sat down?"

"You look comfortable. May I join you?"

"Hello. I brought some ice cream. Would you help me eat it?"

"Do you like chocolate?" (Of course, you need to bring some chocolate with you.)

"Hi, Judy. I brought you something special."

What triggers their memory is not what we say, but what we put in their hands. What they touch, see, smell, and hear helps them connect with their memories. Every time you visit put "something" in their hands:

* Something to share: a flower, variety of garden seeds, a present, postcards, pictures…

* Something to smirk over: a love letter, a book of jokes, a silly mystery item, a funny picture…

* Something to nibble: fruit, popcorn, Cheetos, bread 'n' jam…

* Something to play with: a soft bouncy ball, a balloon to bat, a noodle to swat heinies that walk by, two squirt guns, bubbles to blow…

* Something to hear (bring headphones): birds singing, familiar songs, their favorite person's or a child's voice, a Broadway or radio show…

* Something to smell: lilacs, bacon, cinnamon rolls, lotion…

Bringing my mom a small gift makes us friends instantly, but it gets expensive. So I sneak something from my mom's room, take it home, wrap it, and gift it again.

On Mother's Day, I took my mother something special from her past, her mother's purse. It was a small, beaded, cloth handbag filled with keepsakes that belonged to her mother (who died at a young age, but memories still lingered on in spite of my mom's Alzheimer's). When Mom opened the clasp of the handbag, she found several things inside that she could take out and hold in her hands—tiny gloves, fancy combs that were used in her mother's hair, a ring box with an opal ring, a small envelope and a note inside with her mother's handwriting, and a small portrait of her mother and father.

Very carefully, she took out everything; very carefully she put back everything. She smiled as she did it. She enjoyed smelling and touching everything. For a long time, Mom sat at the table and enjoyed the purse. She laid each thing on the table while we talked about her mother. Her favorite memory was seeing her mother brush her long brown hair as she stood in her bedroom in front of the mirror. She brushed it and then arranged it on the top of her head using the combs to keep it in place. —Excerpt from Butterscotch Sundaes: My Mom's Story of Alzheimer's by Virginia McCone

Family heirlooms and keepsakes are irreplaceable. If you leave them in a memory care community they will be misplaced, or hidden. Create a moment of joy by bringing them with you to visit, then take them home again. Stuff isn't valuable until it brings a smile to someone's face.

If you didn't bring "something" and sense they are struggling, take the pressure off by talking in ways that don't require a response.

"This weekend I went to…"
"The weather today is…"
"I talked with your sister and she…"
"At church the pastor talked about…"
"I've got a dog named and he is…"
"My daughter is…"
"You're such a good mom because…"
"When I was a kid we used to…"

Don't feel like you have to stay for a long period of time. The length of time is irrelevant; it's the quality of time that counts. (Where have you heard that one?)

A "good visit" can be a word that comes out completely wrong, leaving both of us exploding in uncontrollable laughter. —SHARON SNIR, SYDNEY, AUSTRALIA

Don't think you have to "talk" to create a moment. If the person no longer has words, visit without words.

* A bowl of strawberries
* A picture of a train and a train whistle on an iPhone
* An iPad with a video of your pet or their pet
* A makeup bag to beautify
* Old postcards to reminisce
* A video of a kid's baseball game (bring the kid, too)
* Old hats; a silly bow tie
* A "treasure" from the attic
* A "treat" from your pocket

While you are visiting, acknowledge the other people who live there as if they are your friends (which eventually they will be). Be inclusive: bring chocolate for everyone; have a tea party for everyone. Create camaraderie. Better yet, take a few minutes and share the fond memories and fun facts you know about this person with everyone.

They feel your presence more than your words. Just your being there brings joy. And practice, practice, practice. You will get better at visiting each time you go.

We as humans have the incredible ability to breathe life into the ones around us…What an incredible honor and responsibility. —JASMARINA WALSHIRE

Newfound "Something"

Let's Talk Communication

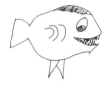

Throughout this book, I make it sound like people with Alzheimer's are talking, but most of the time I am simply interpreting what someone is saying by listening with all of my senses. Listen beyond the words, which is essentially what they are doing, too. Ninety percent of what they understand is not the words coming out of your mouth, it's your body language and tone of voice. You speak volumes without a single word.

Tips to improve communication
* Try a calm, matter-of-fact demeanor.
* Visit in a quiet space away from noise.
* Have a one-on-one conversation; three people talking is too hard for them to follow.
* Use positive body language and facial expressions.
* Position yourself directly in front of the person at eye level and get their attention before speaking.
* Touch the person on the shoulder, knee, or hand to make your presence known.
* Say their name.
* Demonstrate with actions and words.
* Speak slowly in a low-pitched voice.
* Use familiar simple words in short sentences.
* Talk in a pleasant manner.
* Avoid pronouns: "He went…" "She said…" Instead: "Tom went…" "Judy said…"
* Ask yes/no questions: "Would you like some tea?"(while holding a teacup).
* Listen to their tone of voice and body language.

* Take out "don't," "remember" and "no."
* Avoid questions that require short-term memory: "Did your son come to see you today?"
* Access the person's long-term memory: "John is a wonderful son."
* Don't talk over, through, or about them as if they aren't there. They can hear, think, and feel emotions!
* Give simple instructions one step at a time. (The task of brushing teeth contains eleven steps.)
* Praise with a hug, a smile, or a pat on the back.
* If you aren't getting through, walk away and try again later.

When we drive by the care community, my little guy, Keegan, says, "Let's go see the peoples." When children visit be sure to give them something to share. On this visit my little guy had a new pair of cowboy boots. I knew that would create a moment.

When we walked in, a new gentleman motioned my little guy to come over to him. Keegan showed off his boots. The gentleman said, "Wow! Whoa!" Then Keegan stood on one foot. The gentleman said, "Wow! Whoa!" Then Keegan spun around in a circle. The gentleman said, "Wow! Whoa!" I whispered into Keegan's ear, "Ask him what his name is." Keegan asked. The gentleman couldn't tell us his name, but he made my little guy feel special in a matter of a moment. Who does my little guy want to visit? The gentleman who only says, "Wow! Whoa!"

These two gentlemen taught me more about communication in a moment than I learned in a lifetime. I could talk and talk for twelve hours if someone would let me. But when we talk and talk, all they hear is "Wah, wah, wah." It may only take a few words to make someone feel heard, like, "Wow" and "Whoa."

When I affirm my dad's conversation, whether I understand it or not, we are more likely to go into a meaningful conversation that I do understand. —A son's advice

---

Newfound "Wow...Whoa"

Quality Connections

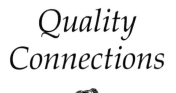

Walking down the hall, you say "Hi!" to the first person, "How are ya?" to the second, and "Good to see ya!" (with a pat on the shoulder) to the third. Despite your good intentions, you are actually causing confusion. The first person is still sleeping. The second person is really nice and responds, "Does someone need me. Who was that?" The third person is thinking, "Who just hit me?" If you cannot make a quality connection, be as quiet as a church mouse as you pass by.

A quality connection means to stop, get down to their eye level, touch their knee, make eye contact, and compliment, compliment, compliment. "Joe, I love that hat on you." "Alice, I wish you would teach me how to sew" (while placing something she has sewn in her lap). "Margaret, did you just get your hair done?" Margaret's hair may be messy, but she doesn't have a mirror. Compliment the person on an attribute that they like about themselves.

"John, you can fix about anything."
"How's my fisherman today?"
"I planted yellow roses, like the ones you love."
"I heard you are a beautiful dancer" (then twirl in your dress).
"I have been bragging 'bout your rhubarb pie."
"Jim, you are a charmer."
"Sally, you make me smile."

Direct statements leave the door wide open for more conversation without putting the person on the spot. They can simply smile back because you made a comment; you didn't ask a question.

Complimenting a lady, I said, "Your cheeks are so rosy." Without missing a beat she replied in a whisper, "Rouge, Dear." Of course, she created two big smiles.

I walked up to a lady whom I didn't know, picked up her hand, and said, "Wow, you have really large hands for a lady." She beamed and replied, "Cause I did a man's work."

Replace "You were…" with "You are…" Even though they no longer sew, they are still an accomplished seamstress. Even though they no longer sail the ocean, they are still the Captain. Remind them who they are and give them their memories back. It takes thirty seconds.

Close your eyes…and go back…waaaaay back: I'm talking about hide and seek at dusk back…
  * *Hot bread and butter.*
  * *Penny candy in a brown bag.*
  * *Hopscotch, kickball, and "Annie-I-Over!"*
  * *When around the corner seemed far away.*
  * *And going downtown seemed like going somewhere.*
  * *Climbing trees.*
  * *Building forts.*
  * *Licking the beaters when your mom made a cake.*
  Didn't it feel good…just to go back and say, "Yeah, I remember that!" That's a quality connection.

A candle loses nothing lighting another candle. —JAMES KELLER

Newfound Connection

Yes 'n' No Questions

We tend to ask open-ended questions like, "What did you do today?" This requires them to remember and talk in a complete sentence. Both are difficult. It's our responsibility to turn our questions around so all they have to say is yes or no. "Are you a farmer?" "Are you a businessman?" You know by the light in their eyes whether you hit something or missed something. If there is very little response, try a general statement like, "I bet you are a hard worker."

Richard would walk up and down the halls repeating, "I'm hungry, I'm hungry, I'm hungry." I asked him, "What do you like to eat?" He just kept repeating, "I'm hungry, I'm hungry." Reminding myself of this tool, I said, "Do you like warm chocolate chip cookies?" He stopped, "Yes." "Do you like chicken?" He said, "No." "Do you like roast with potatoes?" He said, "Uh huh." "Do you like pasta?" He said, "Could live without it." "Do you like carrots?" "Yeah." The list went on and on and by the end I knew exactly what he liked and didn't like. At supper that night he would not sit down and eat. Guess what was for supper…chicken and pasta.

What NOT to say: "What did you do this morning?" "What did you have for lunch?" "Remember the drive I took you on yesterday?" "How are your kids?" "Did you have a good weekend?" "Do you remember…?"

What TO say: "You got your hair done this morning." "Are you hungry?" "Would you like to go for a drive?" "Sally, your youngest, is smart like you." "I had such a good weekend. Did you?" "I remember when…"

The heart is for making life choices; the mind is for deciding whether to choose a spoon or a fork. —MICHAEL BILLINGTON

Newfound Question

"How Are You?"

When you ask, "How are you?," you are asking the person to respond with words, which can be difficult. Or they have to look at how they really feel: "My stomach hurts. I don't feel so good. Will you call my daughter?," which takes you fifteen minutes to resolve. Instead…

* Compliment them…"Love your hair today."
* Say, "Good mornin', Sunshine!"
* Take their hands 'n' say, "So good to see you!"
* Stick out your tongue 'n' tease them: "Hey, Sassy!"
* Lightly embrace: "May I give you a kiss on the cheek?"
* Wink at them: "Hello, Sweetheart!"
* Roll your eyes 'n' make a funny face.
* Rub/scratch their back.
* Bend down 'n' smile.
* Sneak "something" from your pocket.
* Play peek-a-boo.
* Whisper a secret.

How can you make someone feel better, in a matter of a moment?

When we were little and visited my grandpa, we would say, "How ya feeling, Grandpa?" He would reply with a smile, "With my fingers." As he grew older, he lost his ability to respond verbally. But one day I said, "How ya feeling, Grandpa?" And to my amazement, he replied, "With my fingers."

—A GRANDDAUGHTER

There are, however, those who possess a wealth of merriment which spills out of the pockets of their souls. —TERESA COSTELLO, S.P.

Newfound Merriment

When In Doubt...Laugh

If you are having a bad day—maybe your co-worker or a family member is frustrating you—you can still do this:

Go into the person's room and say with a smile, "My co-worker is driving me crazy. I hope she is gone tomorrow." Laugh deeply. "Your boy, who lives in Alabama, thinks he is so smart." Laugh deeply. "My husband is a jerk. He'd better not come home tonight." Laugh deeply. As long as you laugh and have a smile on your face, you pretty much can say whatever it is you are thinking. Remember, 90 percent of what they understand is not your words. What they understand is your body language, facial expressions, and tone of voice. So laugh and get out your frustrations, but plant a smile on your face.

Laughing enhances our sense of well-being, reduces stress, and improves our ability to survive a crisis. Physically, it increases circulation, reduces blood pressure, promotes brain functioning, relaxes muscles, reduces pain by increasing endorphins in the bloodstream, and stimulates the thymus gland, which improves the immune system.

I know that information isn't funny, but hopefully it helps you understand the power of laughter. If you laugh a lot, when you are older all your wrinkles will be in the right places.

Alzheimer's has robbed Mother of her memories, not her heart. Her sense of humor is alive and well. Although some of her brightness is vanishing, we are making new memories every day and we are still laughing a lot.

If you haven't noticed, people with dementia can make incredibly witty and funny comments. I used to keep a small book in which I wrote down the funny things they did and said. This book was read by all, and yes it created laughter.

Surround yourself with things that make you laugh: jokes, funny cards, comic strips, fun "stuff." Arrive at someone's bedside with a joke instead of complaining about your day.

A caregiver who liked to tell jokes told me that when she told jokes to people with dementia they would roar with laughter, even if they didn't understand. It was all about the inflection in her voice and beginning the joke with a familiar phrase, such as "Did you hear the one about...?"

Whatever it takes to laugh, do it! You will be healthier for it and so will the people around you. I love it when someone's laugh is funnier than the joke.

Luey: Sam, you know the worst thing about growing old?
Sam: No...what's that? Luey: What's what?

Newfound Funny

Share Your Life

When you have a few minutes, share your life: getting married, having a baby, or a weekend adventure. Bring pictures and videos and share your story.

> I went to the ocean last week. We walked out on this jetty. The wind blew so hard it crashed the waves against the rocks. The ice blue water tasted salty—like eating salt straight out of the container. I could see fishing boats and then they would be gone behind these enormous waves. I took off my shoes and walked along the beach, picking up broken shells. The water was so cold, it numbed my feet. There was a deep-red-colored starfish on one of the larger rocks. It was absolutely beautiful. —JOLENE

Avoid talking about financial stresses, someone being sick, or someone dying, because that feeling you created will linger on after you leave. But absolutely share anything and everything that brings you joy.

> A week after I had my first child, I brought her in and let the residents hold her. A staff member asked, "Aren't you afraid they might drop her?" I said, reassuringly, "It will be okay." Angela, in the latest stage of Alzheimer's, held her, perked up, then said clearly, "Beautiful baby." They loved touching her little fingers. As she grew, I placed her in the middle of the living room and let her play for all to see. They gave me a gift with their smiling faces. Still today my daughter feels very comfortable with older people. The gift goes both ways.

A good story—like a grand old waltz—takes us from our immediacy and gives us a chance to regroup, reform, and re-enter the dance of life. A good story denies universal defeat and so gives us a glimpse of ultimate joy. —SISTER TERESA, S.P.

Newfound Story

Magic Words

W hen you are really upset, isn't it wonderful to have a friend to call who knows just what to say or can make you laugh? When a person with dementia is troubled, here are some magic words:

"I will be here all day."
"Don't worry. I'll take care of it."
"If you need anything, just let me know."
"I do silly things like that, too."
"Between the two of us, we will be okay."
"You are pretty special."
"Wow, you are so smart!"
"Thank you. I couldn't have done it without you."
"That's a good idea. I'll have to try that!"
"You always look out for me."
"Hey, Ornery! Are you staying out of trouble?"
"Hello, Handsome!"

When he is confused and it's causing him frustration, I lighten him instantly with, "Have you been boozin' today?" —NUTTY CAREGIVER

When my lady starts to get upset I softly run my fingers through her hair. Calms her right down. —A CAREGIVER

Simply listening can be magical.

Modern science is trying to produce a tranquilizer more effective than a few kind words. —UNKNOWN

Newfound Magic Words

Saying Goodbye

S aying goodbye is never easy, but hopefully I can make it easier. When you are getting close to departing, start to make comments that leave the person with positive feelings. Feelings of assurance, feelings of self-worth, and feelings of love.

> "Can I visit you again?"
> "I really enjoyed talking with you."
> "I enjoyed your company so much. This has been lovely."
> "I haven't laughed this hard in a long time. Thank you."
> "Let's pray before I go."
> "Your smile always makes my day."
> "I need to use the bathroom. I'll be right back."

You don't have to be right back. You don't even have to come back at all. If you're going to be gone until tomorrow or next week, give them the hope you will be back soon. You can walk out the door and walk back in and they will say, "Where have you been?" Give them a place they don't want to go: "I need to go to work, but I'll see you soon." "I have to go to the dentist to get my tooth pulled. Will you pray for me?" Avoid saying, "I have to go home," because that will trigger them to want to go home.

When leaving, give them hugs, reassuring touches, and a smile. The bottom line is, if you're cheerful the person will be more comfortable with you leaving.

Never say goodbye, because goodbye means going away and going away means forgetting. —J. M. BARRIE, PETER PAN

Newfound "See Ya Soon!"

Sparking Moments

When I say, "I'd lose my head if it wasn't attached," I think of my mother, who said it often. When you see a certain flower, you think of a certain person. When you feel silky pink satin, you remember your prom dress.

Joan and Ray met at a singles group. Ray asked Joan what she thought of the group: "There's just a bunch of losers here." They started dating and eventually got married. Faithfully, twice a year, Ray sent Joan a dozen roses "From the loser." Ray was diagnosed with Alzheimer's before the age of fifty-two. Joan kept him at home for a long time. One day while grocery shopping, Ray wandered off. When she found him, he was in the flower department. He stated, "Want buy." "You want to buy some roses?," she asked. He nodded. The next morning he walked into the kitchen and questioned the roses. "You bought them for me last night." She saw a light in his eye: "Oh yeah, they are from the loser." She cried. Not moments later he was "gone" again. Roses opened the window to his memory for a moment.

A basketball coach who had Parkinson's went into a coma. His family said what "brought him back" was when everyone began addressing him as "Coach" while putting his hands on a basketball.

When my mom had a major stroke, she couldn't figure out how to raise her arms. I told her to block the shot (she was a guard in basketball, six on six). She responded instantly.

—Wendie Fagan

Alzheimer's cannot take away what had already been. It only transfers the responsibility of remembering to those who love the one who is afflicted. —Natasha, in a letter to her grandfather

Newfound Spark

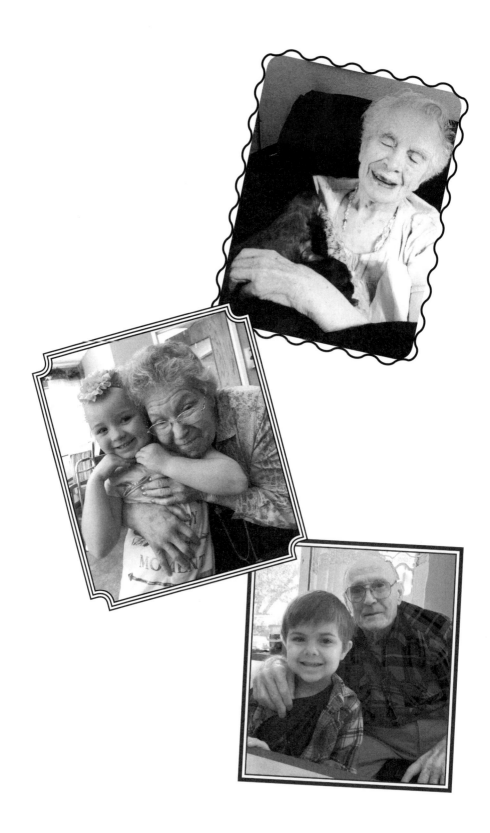

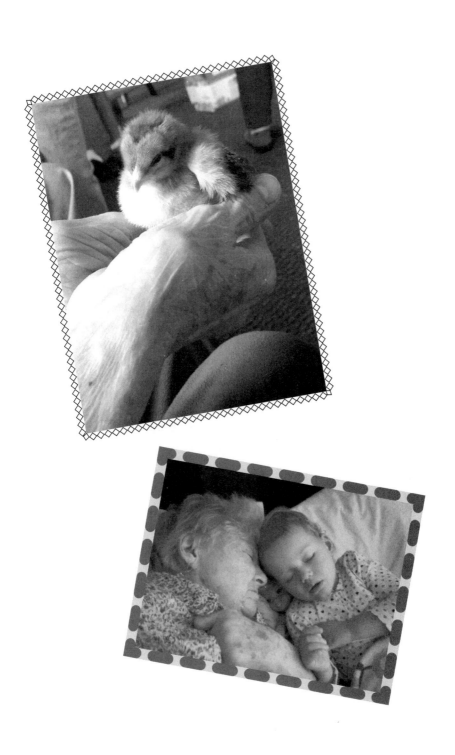

Art vs. Crafts

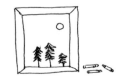

Blessed is the person who gives a person with dementia a blank paper to create whatever shows up in the space. Be sure the person can see the edges, whether those edges are black lines or a midrange-colored paper behind the white paper. Pull them out of the darkness by placing "something familiar" for them to see—for example, a picture of a windmill, a significant place, a beloved pet, a flower, a child, a tree, a sunset, or a bird. The possibilities are limitless. Allow them to express their emotions and memory through color. Or give them a chunk of clay to feel with their fingers and manipulate however they choose. That is art.

I brought in art materials to create a decoration for my sister's door. It was a great project that was fun for us both. After we hung it on the door, she told me, "Thank you. I will never forget you."

Simply let them look upon artwork of all genres and ask them, "What do you see?," or, "How does this painting make you feel?" The part of the brain that governs feelings and what they see is still very much intact. If a certain painting doesn't draw them out, continue to change the art they see. Different art speaks to different people.

When there are expectations or step-by-step instructions to get a certain outcome, we are setting them up to fail. When staff is making it, that is a craft.

Residents were asked to take old greeting cards, fold them in thirds, and put a little ribbon at the top to make bookmarks. Guess what they were doing with the greeting cards? Unfolding them and reading them, at which point staff corrected again and again and said, "No, keep it folded. We are making bookmarks." What do we do with greeting cards? Read them.

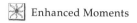

Quilting or cutting out patterns and fabrics simply works! At what age did they learn to cut? Four. Their body remembers. And, yes, sharp scissors, especially for quilters. Some think, "They can't have sharp scissors!" Is it possible that we keep them so safe we take away their joys? Let this person be your teacher about whether or not they can cut with sharp scissors. They may not be able to quilt with a tiny needle, but they can take the fabrics they've cut out and arrange them on a quilting square.

Engaging in a task their body has done for a lifetime is stronger than any medication. It slows down the breathing, reduces agitation, and brings life back into their being because they are stimulated in a way that is beyond words. Even if they haven't painted or written poetry, when you give space for all things to show up, it will be beautiful.

The Master once proposed a riddle: "What do the artist and the musician have in common with the mystic?" Everyone gave up. "The realization that the finest speech does not come from the tongue." —ANTHONY DE MELLO

Newfound Art

"Help Me"

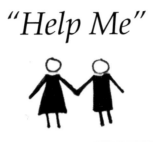

Whatever your task may be, ask the person to help you. Human beings possess an innate desire to be needed. Encouraging them to be responsible for the home might make it seem more like "home."

> *Overcaring can diminish independence and self worth. I see so much pride from a person when they make their bed. Too often our helpful hearts want to do for them tasks we see as mundane, but when we allow them to live their life and participate in every corner of their life fully—even the mundane—we have given joy-purpose-connection. If we squash any one of those—joy-purpose-connection—we start down the slippery slope of depression and dependence. (By the way, making the bed maintains balance and range of motion and other good stuff in a normal way!)*
>
> —Natalie Kunkel, dementia expert

People need to be needed, no matter what their age or their physical or mental ability. If the person taught English, ask her to edit a paper or help a younger person with their homework. If they fixed cars, describe the noise coming from your car and give them the opportunity to tell you what they think it is. If they had children, ask for advice on discipline. If they were a doctor or nurse, describe some symptoms and get their diagnosis. And, who knows, the advice they give you will probably work.

Have them help you clean a closet, cut out coupons, move boxes, sweep the patio, rake leaves, hang clothes, wipe furniture, wash dishes, fold laundry, peel oranges and eggs, sort cards, stack wood, shell corn to feed the squirrels, water the garden, snap beans, clean strawberries, polish and sort silverware, crack peanuts, tear lettuce, butter bread, and on 'n' on.

Create chores that don't even need to be done. The key is to choose something they have done frequently in the past. However they help you, let them know, "Thank you! I could not have done that without you." You can offer the same projects every day because they don't remember they did it the day before.

Once a week I would pull out a box of yarn, unroll it, and bring it into the living room and say, "I found this in the closet, and it's a mess. Would you help me roll it up?" Men helped, too, because they liked to help the ladies. If someone looked blankly at the yarn I would put my hand over hers and kick-start the motion.

We would put a few dishes in the sink, squirt them with ketchup, and ask a lady to help with the dishes.

Lug a suitcase into a room like you just "found" it in the attic. "I wonder what is in here? Will you help me unpack this suitcase?"

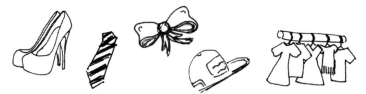

Be silly 'n' play dress-up. Give them the hope that they will "travel the world someday."

When you ask the person to help you weed the garden, they may pull up flowers or pick veggies not quite ready. The point is…their fingers are in the dirt. And together you can make mud pies for dessert.

☼ Never look down on anybody unless you are helping them up. —Jesse Jackson

---

Newfound Play

Drink Up

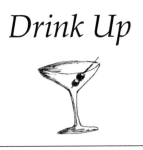

When a person is dehydrated, what happens? Increased confusion, urinary tract infection, constipation, incontinence, decreased metabolism, headaches, daytime fatigue, intensified arthritis, pain, decreased functioning, and they're more likely to fall. Who suffers the repercussions? You. So let's talk about ways to get someone to drink up!

It isn't enough to just place a pitcher of water beside their bed or a cup of water in front of them. A person with dementia often loses their sense of thirst or is unable to tell you when they're thirsty. Again, apply the concept that they only know what they see. You're more likely to create thirst by pouring ice-cold water in front of them and saying, "I'm parched!," or, "Let's wet our whistles!," or even, "It's sure hot today," and drink with them.

No one particularly loves water, so find out what drink they do love and make it resemble that. Lemonade in a martini glass, apple juice in a whiskey bottle, or grape juice in a wine glass. Pour water into see-through colored glasses so it becomes Kool-Aid. Pour liquid into a McDonald's cup with a lid and straw to pretend it's soda. If water doesn't taste right, try adding herbs or sliced fruits.

A husband knew his wife liked vodka, so he put water in shot glasses and they would "take shots" together.

While singing, I brought out a pitcher of water with little red cups. I commented how parched I was, and as I went around the room some people declined the water. But a beautiful thing happened when I made a second pass. The people who declined the first time were now accepting the offer. I attributed the success to their seeing others drink up.

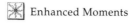

Serve warm liquids in the morning to increase their metabolism and offer liquids frequently during the day. Of course, they will want coffee, coffee, and coffee…and thirty seconds after they drink their coffee, they will want another cup. Use their short-term memory loss to your advantage by saying over and over again, "The coffee is brewing. The coffee is brewing." Caffeine dehydrates people, so serve decaffeinated coffee diluted with water.

Pick your battles. If they grow upset because you won't give them more coffee, and they refuse water or other liquids, by all means let them enjoy their coffee. Consider that a "night cap" is warmer to the soul than any medication.

Uncle Jo was so drunk he hung himself over the back of the chair and put his pants to bed. —JYOTI

Newfound Drink

Walking,
Walking, Walking

Walking, walking, walking does wonders. It relieves stress, it allows for a good night's rest or a nap, and it helps strengthen their leg muscles so they are less likely to fall. Because this person is younger in their mind, they are more mobile than most older people. When you hear about elderly ladies jumping over a fence without even tearing their skirts, now you'll know why—they are sixteen all over again!

> *My wife was very restless. She would pace from one end to the other of our dead-end street for over an hour. She didn't want me to walk with her, so I just let her go. I set a lawn chair on the sidewalk and watched her until she got tired. She no longer does this; some things get better.* —Paul Edwards

Pacing, pacing, pacing is common. Many wish for a magic potion to give this person peace of mind. Sometimes it's just not possible. Pacing may be the only way to ease the moment. Usually they pace because they are unable to calm themselves down. What would be a reason they understand to sit down? Coffee? Ice cream? How can you help "ground" them? Wrapping them up; giving them a hot wet washcloth; placing your hand heavily on their knee or shoulder, or a rice bag over their lap. Or, simply let them walk, walk, walk to wear themselves out. My mama says, "When you can't fix it, go for a walk."

> *At 3:00 every day, Lindel, age sixty, would become upset and want to "get out of here." If we ignored him, it would get worse. I became proactive. At 1:30 every afternoon I would gather up people and go for a stroll. The more we walked, the better the day went. If Lindel was beyond calming I would say, "I need to get out of here, too! Let me grab my coat." I would*

tell someone where I hoped to go and to come look for us if we weren't back in an hour.

When we started walking, I let him have an "illusion of control" by asking, "Which way should we go?" Lindel usually chose the same direction every time—away from traffic and toward residential homes. While walking the first block, I let him vent his anger. At the corner, depending on this mood, I still gave him the illusion of control by again asking, "Now which way should we go?" Walking down the next block I would talk about his "greatness": fishing and his kids. "How many kids do you have?" "Boys or girls?" "Do you like to fish?" Do you catch walleye? Pike? Perch?"

When we came to the next corner I would again ask, "Which way should we go?" And while Lindel was deciding I would innocently say, "I think this way looks good. What do you think?" (illusion of choice). Because he didn't know where we were, he usually agreed with me. I would notice things like nature, a pretty house, or the weather. The main purpose was to get his mind off his perceived problems and get him to like me. When we got to the next corner, I would try to head back toward the community by saying, "You know what? I think I recognize something down this street. Let's go this way." On good days, we walked right back into the community by my saying, "My feet hurt. I would like rest and get a drink here." On other days, we walked two miles in the rain.

Although Lindel was difficult, he was a blessing. Because of him, we started a walking program in which everyone benefited. People relaxed more, chair and bed alarms did not exist, and people were walking till they passed.

On these walks I would purposefully take people in wheelchairs because those who had difficulty walking could hang onto the side of the wheelchair. Pearl, one of the better walkers, would push a separate wheelchair. If Therstin walked too far ahead, I didn't say, "Therstin, come back here!," because then he thinks someone is after him. I said, "Hey, wait up for us!" In other words, be a gentleman.

So often caregivers are afraid to open the door because the person might run away. From my experience, when you open the door, they walk ten feet, don't know where they are, and ask for assistance.

I don't recommend that just anyone goes on these walks. It takes a person who is comfortable because they can sense insecurity. If you're secure and going on these walks, please bring along a bag of goodies for snacking along the way.

I "lost" two people when I worked in memory care. Therstin being one of them. One day I went in the building for just a moment and when I came back out, he was gone. He was found two hours later in an apartment complex nearby. The other person was Pearl. She snuck out the window and was found lounging on a back patio next door. They are mobile, but this doesn't mean you stop going for walks. It means you have to know these people. But even if you do, life happens. It doesn't mean you seal your windows shut. It just means that they only open one quarter of the way so people cannot sneak through.

In addition to walking, we had an exercise routine every morning and physical activities throughout the day (sweeping the patio or clearing the tables).

> *I just want to share this thought that lies heavily on my heart. Perhaps it will help someone else. As John's pace slowed, I didn't change mine. One day as we were walking up a small hill he asked, "Why do you always walk ahead of me?" Even today, the memory hurts. May we catch what we are doing before it becomes a sad memory.*
>
> —JOAN

Let me explain how wandering paths came about. In nursing homes there are long hallways with no place to sit. They see the door at the end of the hallway, and in the hope of going home they head toward it, but when they get there it's locked. Turning around, they see the door at the other end of the hallway...Hence, they are labeled as "wandering." Our environments have caused many "behaviors."

We then created environments with racetracks/wandering paths going around multipurpose areas so we could see everyone. The problem is that the people who live here can also see and hear everyone. Research clearly shows that the person with Alzheimer's cannot handle lots of people and large spaces. Now they can see/hear someone yelling, they can see/hear someone crying, they can see/hear someone who "wants out." Now you have people escalated in their dementia because they are bouncing off of (reacting to) everything they see and hear.

Yes, it may be impossible for this person to walk alone, but walk with them in dignity! "I am going for a walk. Would you like to join me?"

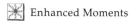

A clever occupational therapist purposefully showed her cleavage to get men to escort her down the hall. In another instance, I watched a young male occupational therapist use a belt to help a lady walk and asked her to count to ten as she walked. You should have seen the look of contempt she gave that boy for insulting her abilities.

They will also walk better with a steady beat or marching, because that is what they did in the classroom as children.

Dorothy shuffled around, mumbling noises to herself; but when someone started singing "I've Been Working on the Railroad," she piped right up singing every word, stood up straighter, and shuffled less.

They are giving you the opportunity to show them you respect their wishes, you respect their right to make decisions, and you love the essence of who they are. Be glad of the opportunity. —CLAUDIA STRAUSS

Newfound Path

Quiet as a
Church Mouse

When a person is connecting with someone or something, your job is to be as quiet as a church mouse. When you're talking in the background, you walk by quickly, or you create a loud noise, their attention will go to you. They could have been reminiscing about tipping over outhouses as a prank, but the connection to that memory will be gone in a second.

Noise is the number one reason connections and activities fail:

* Medications can wait.
* Asking someone if they have to use the bathroom can wait.
* Telling your co-worker something can wait.
* Your thought can wait.
* Answering your cell phone can wait.

Be as quiet as a church mouse…during the church service, during an activity, during entertainment, and during a meal. Whatever you think you have to do can wait until the connection is complete.

A talented guitar player was singing and a gentleman was all smiles as he watched and listened. Then a medication aide bent down in front of him blocking his view of the entertainer. Frustration on his face, he waved his hand, motioning for her to move. She tried and tried to get him to take his medication. He refused and was now upset. She came back later with his medication mixed with "chocolate something," and still he pushed her away. This went on in the middle of an activity that everyone was trying to enjoy. Not only was he upset, but the other residents were distracted by the commotion this med aide put into motion. Who needs to change?

"Being with someone" is more important than any medication or anything we think we "have to do." It's not about what is on the calendar. It is about creating space for residents, families, and caregivers to do what they love here.

Quiet means there is no phone ringing in the background. The ringing will interrupt your connections, again causing activities to fail. Place the phone where they can't see it or hear it, or change the ring tone so it doesn't sound like a phone.

While we were singing the old familiar songs, the phone rang in the background and three got up to answer it.

In the memory care community create a quiet space, even if you have to convert a storage space. In this space is a couch to nap on, afghans to wrap up in, lotion, soothing music, stuffed animals, warm hats/gloves, rice bags to warm in the microwave, hot wet washcloths with scents of lavender, and hands that touch with great care. Maybe there is even an old-style hairdryer so they can hunker under the heat as the world goes away. When anyone is going "over the top" because of too much noise and stimulation, simply let them rest in a quiet space away from the world.

Silence is like rich sensuous water after a long trek in the desert. —Donna Bulter, S.P.

Newfound Silence

Breaking of Bread

Written by Teresa Stecker, R.N., Pastor. (P.S., She's my sister.)

One of the most powerful and common rituals symbolizing Christian faith is communion, or the Lord's Supper. Not only is it an outward indication of Christian faith, it is one that has been significant since the early years of a person's religious training. Communion for Christian believers is an outward expression of worship to indicate their union with Jesus Christ and with His body, the church. It has been described as a love feast with the Savior, the language of our soul.

The Lord Jesus, on the night he was betrayed, took bread, and when he had given thanks, he broke it and said, "This is my body, which is for you; do this in remembrance of me." In the same way, after supper he took the cup, saying, "This cup is the new covenant in my blood; do this, whenever you drink it, in remembrance of me" (1 Corinthians 11:23-25 NIV in the Christian Holy Book, the Bible).

Our Protestant church has a nursing home ministry to four care centers, including one memory care community. As the Lenten season approached, we rediscovered the significance of communion offered to all believers. Little did we realize the impact of this hour of providing communion to our eighty nursing home residents. Besides our Christian beliefs about communion, our goal in bringing communion to these residents was to demonstrate that they are needed, honored, indispensable, and dignified as members of the body of Christ. (See 1 Corinthians 12.)

We wanted to reach all of their senses. To create the feeling of church, we incorporated several people in the communion, including church members, family members, and staff. Even if they did not partake, their presence suggested a church.

We asked church members to dress up in their Sunday best and our pastor to wear his typical attire for a communion service.

We set up a table draped with linen, placed a vase full of roses, and lit candles to create the look and feel of a sanctuary. All the while, hymns were playing in the background. We spent time physically preparing participants by combing hair, adjusting clothes, and helping with other personal grooming. We prepared each one spiritually through prayer, scripture reading, or conversation regarding the significance of sharing the sacrament of the Lord's Supper. We selected scripture that has personal significance and familiarity. With communion, we assisted with the receiving of elements. If they were unable to physically drink or eat the bread and wine, we touched the elements to their lips. We prayed individually with each one present and then concluded with corporate recitation of the Lord's Prayer. After the communion, we finished with an act of blessing by giving them a rose, touching their arm, and affirming their value as a member of the body of Christ.

We also served communion in individual rooms, and it included the same elements of our group communion. The response of the residents was incredible and powerful. It created a solemn and sacred time. In an environment that can be noisy and chaotic, there was an attitude of reverence by all present. After receiving communion, an emotional eighty-year-old woman said she had felt the church had forgotten her—until this day. An elderly gentleman wept as we held his hand and prayed for his physical health. A wheelchair-bound person indicated that this was the best day of her life in the care center. As church members, we felt honored and blessed to bring a significant and joyful moment to those individuals with Alzheimer's disease.

We sensed the gratitude of all who participated. This included a wife who indicated that she was in church with her husband for the first time in more than two years. They shared songs, communion side-by-side, and the Lord's Prayer. They had this moment to reconnect with each other, their faith, and their God.

If communion is not happening, families can go to their church leaders and request it. Connection with the church and its rituals is relevant in creating spiritual well-being.

☼ It is understood that we are all saved. If not,
you misunderstood. —Sister Ruth, S.P.

Newfound Prayer

Final
Moments

Look beyond the wall of this disease and focus
on the person who needs you. Love and care with
a genuine heart. That's when you will fly, feel
warmth, and start smelling the daisies. —JOLENE

Windows in the Brain

"Soft music" was how I communicated with and cared for my first friend, a friend I met when my new husband, Jim, and I moved to his hometown. A knock at the door and what was to come changed my life regarding how to care for loved ones with Alzheimer's.

The lovely lady at the door was Anna. She had a big smile and a plate of kringla for the newlyweds. Anna began telling me that she was Jim's Sunday school teacher and that she loved him, too…Hmmm, I thought. She asked me if I liked to sing. "Yes, I do." She then asked, "Are you a soprano?" I said yes. She smiled. "We'll be the canaries together in the church choir."

Later in her years Anna's demeanor was noticeably changing, and her daughter came to live with her. I took a couple of years off from work, and when I returned Anna was there. She didn't know me, and I wasn't familiar with what I was about to encounter. Anna was hostile and not nice at all. I sobbed and the nurse explained to me a little about Alzheimer's. Days and weeks went by as I learned to accept Anna as she was now. I smiled and spoke softly every chance I could. I was assigned to give Anna her bath, which I observed was not pleasant. But I said a little prayer for us and proceeded. I warmed her chair and gently sprayed warm water first on her legs and slowly moved upward. She began to get upset, so I decided to sing softly, "I Love to Tell The Story," a song she had sung many times at church. Much to my surprise, she started singing with me in perfect pitch. I got to her shoulder and then her hair. She jerked and went one octave higher in perfect pitch still. We finished her song and finished her bath—who knew! After that I did Anna's bath every time, whether I was assigned to her or not. She wasn't always that agreeable, but that was okay. Find out the story of their life before Alzheimer's and introduce it to them every chance you can in a gentle, peaceful way. I love being a CNA.

—FROM THE LOVING HEART OF ROSEMARY BRACKEY

Our brain is full of well-lit, airy, vacant rooms with an open window in each one. Imagine if by the time you are in your sixties, you were to find yourself searching for a thought in the memory room, only to find that the room had become dark, the drapes drawn. That's what happens to a person with Alzheimer's.

One such person was a large-framed, boisterous farmer who spoke with a salty vocabulary. First, the memory room in his brain became dark, then other rooms darkened as they were covered with a black shroud called plaque that continued to spread slowly from room to room. As this happened to the farmer, he became a shell of the man his family and friends once knew. In time, he forgot how to feed himself, had trouble with swallowing, couldn't do his activities of daily living skills, and could barely stand long enough to transfer from the bed to the wheelchair. His face became expressionless, and his eyes stared vacantly. I was sure that most of the windows in his brain had shut, become locked, and would never open again. I was wrong!

You know how the window frame in an old house doesn't fit quite tight, and a small amount of air seeps between the sill and the frame? One evening, I was pushing the farmer's wheelchair and a visitor reached out his hand and patted the farmer's knee.

"Hello," the visitor greeted. "Hello, Bob," the farmer returned in this booming voice. The blank expression on the farmer's face had changed to one of joy at seeing an old friend. "He knows you!," I exclaimed in surprise. "He should," the visitor replied. "We've been friends for years, and we were both on the board of business in town for a long time, weren't we?" "Yes," the farmer answered with gusto.

I could see a calm look of contentment on his face. "We went to a lot of those board meetings together. This is the man who made a lot of the important decisions at the meetings, didn't you?"

Tears welled up in the farmer's eyes as he struggled to grasp memories long forgotten. I hated to see him so sad, so I tried to add a little humor to the conversation. "Oh, sure! Were those important decisions where to get beer afterward?" Both men laughed at my teasing, as the farmer slowly boomed out, "Yes!"

I explained to the visitor that it was the farmer's bedtime so he had to leave. By the time I wheeled the farmer the short distance down the hall into his room and closed the door, his face was expressionless again. His eyes stared vacantly, focused on the closed drapes just like the drapes that closed in his mind.

—Fay Risner

When I was a little girl in church, Don was the smiling gentleman who would tease me. I moved away for eight years, pursuing my life, family, and work. When I returned to visit my "home church," Don was sitting on the other side of the aisle. I walked over, excited to say hi to my old friend. As I did, a look of fear came over his face. He didn't know me, and I was scaring this gentle man with whom I had grown up. As I was walking back the tears rolled. I, an international speaker on Alzheimer's, had been completely unaware of the sadness that would overtake me when someone I had always adored was now afraid of me. This is what it feels like. Compassion seeped in for every family member and friend of someone with Alzheimer's. I had been making it sound easy, but when someone you love is now afraid of you, it no longer feels like a rose but a thorn. Later in the year, I went back to my church. Don was there but I didn't go up to him. I sang my dad's favorite song, "Go Light Your World," as I have done so often before. I could see Don's smile from way in the back; he was a bright light. When I finished, I walked by him, and I could tell he knew me then. I hugged him with all of me and he told me I sounded like an angel. Tears still well up simply in the telling of my story. —JOLENE

"I miss me," said the lady with Alzheimer's.

Look past your thoughts so you may drink the pure nectar of this Moment. —RUMI

Newfound Window

Late Stages

Just because someone doesn't physically or verbally respond, it doesn't mean they don't feel your presence. With all my heart, I know they are still in there. So continue talking to them, even if they don't talk back. Read to them, touch their cheek, brush their hair, lotion their feet, and imagine you are simply wrapping them up with your love.

> I walked into a dementia community with an administrator and saw a woman shuffling along, muttering noises. The administrator said that she was in her last stages, a typical Alzheimer's person, and that no one was in there. I walked up to that lady and gave her the biggest hug I could give, and she started giggling. Yahooooo!!! I had created a moment of joy. Giggles are far better than nothing at all. Assume there is no one in there, and that's all you will see. Change your attitude and you will find so much more!

I do think there are people who purposefully keep their heads down with their eyes closed, coping the only way they know how. Even people with closed eyes who do not speak can sense the closeness of another person. Let go of your expectations of how you want them to respond and a moment of joy may come when you least expect it.

> A nurse was doing a physical evaluation on a lady in the late stages of dementia. This lady was non-responsive and bedridden. When she began to check the lady's head she felt a huge ridge across her skull. The nurse was startled and said aloud, "What happened there?" The lady piped up as clear as day: "Do you want to hear about that? When I was a child I fell off a stone wall and it cracked my skull. People pampered me because of that." And then she was gone again. The clarity of the lady's words astonished the nurse, but can you imagine how many times she must have told her story? It certainly was not forgotten.

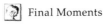

If the person bedbound, paint a mural on the ceiling, hang a mobile, tack up a poster of a baby animal, or hang a kite. Place things outside their window to connect with: a doghouse (no need for the dog), bird feeders, small windmills, wind chimes, a hanging tomato plant, a flowering bush, an old bicycle, a clothesline with sheets blowing in the wind, or the American flag.

I love working with people with dementia. As folks move further into dementia, they often have a childlike innocence about them. I see their souls shining through as their individual identities wane. I meet folks at the heart level, not the head, and that's where I want to be. —KAREN, WHO RADIATES HER HEART

They can sense whether you are comfortable or not, so breathe deeply when you sit with them. Encompass calm, close your eyes with them, and just Be.

We can only know that we know nothing. And that is the highest degree of human wisdom. —LEO TOLSTOY

Newfound Nothing

Power of Touch

Written by Teresa Stecker, R.N., Hospice Nurse, Pastor. (P.S., She's my sister.)

Touch is one of the basic needs of life. The craving for touch to communicate affection, comfort, and reassurance is present the day we enter the world. As a newborn, touch is the first of our senses we use to develop our sense of the world around us. The stroke of a mother's touch calms a baby's cry. As we develop, we seek and welcome meaningful touch through kisses, hugs, playful touch, holding hands, and other positive touches. Touch, like our other senses, gives us clues about the reality around us, our world awareness. It tells us if it is a safe world and a place where we are loved and valued.

Touch that shows anger, anxiety, frustration, and impatience brings tension, agitation, and anxiousness. Touch that shows affection, reassurance, comfort, and value, brings calmness and peace. Touch has the power to break through the feelings you want to transcend. As we age, other senses may change and fade away, but touch remains.

Touch can reach through the fog, confusion, and fear of dementia. Reassuring touch grounds those who are spatially disoriented, brings people back to their bodies, and increases their awareness in present time and space. One touch can affirm that they are not alone and they are valued by the person who is beside them.

We need to stop and think about our touch and what that means to the person, and to those around us who are watching. Your touch may give permission to others to enter an unknown world of dementia. As with the person with dementia, touch can break through the fears of the families. Families may be unsure of what to do, but when they see you touch the person, you are validating that the person is still there. When you do this, families are more likely to move in and do the same thing. Sometimes, our touch of affection isn't so much for the person as it is for the loved one who is watching. It communicates the compassionate and caring part of humanity. Observing powerful touch can completely change the way one thinks about touch.

As Alzheimer's progresses, the critical piece is to find the touch that was meaningful and positive in the person's life. That may be a hug, a kiss, stroking of hair, holding hands, stroking the forearm, touching the forehead (like taking a temperature), or a handshake. It may be dancing or playing "Ring around the Rosie." This touch indicates that you know them because you are touching them in a way in which they are accustomed and comfortable.

In my first two weeks, eighteen residents met my gaze with an icy catatonic glare. I would smile and ask them if they wanted to participate in some new activity. The answer was always the same. The answer was always "No." So I began giving massages. I found myself thinking, if I were in their situation what would I like? A massage would be nice. I brought in bottles of scented oils and lotions. I began rubbing their shoulders, necks, and hands, and as I massaged, I felt their armor fall away. At best, I am a stranger to them. I am not their daughter or a nurse. I am more like a familiar, nameless friend. Sometimes I am "Mrs. Yoo-hoo." Sometimes I am "Hey, hey, hey, you!" No one knows my name. But they know me. They know my spirit. —Sally Dutta

Some would say that touch is personal and not everyone likes to be touched. Too often, we make decisions based upon what we would like. But it's not about us—it is about what the person needs. In my years as a hospice nurse, I have yet to discover someone who refused all forms of touch, especially those alone or without loved ones. It simply comes down to discovering the right way to touch, the kind of touch that brings the most positive response.

In the final days of life, Grace slipped into a semi-coma. In her restlessness, her husband of forty years stroked her cheek and her forearm. Whenever he left the room, he planted a small kiss on her cheek. The family, in unspoken agreement, decided that Grace would know she was not alone by communicating their presence through touch. So, her children and grandchildren took turns holding her hand. In her final days, she looked peaceful—no frown, no agitated movement of extremities, her muscles relaxed and breathing easy. She died peacefully with her son holding her hand. Through the simple and significant acts of touch, Grace felt loved until her last breath.

Our hands—the tools of touch—are powerful. We can hurt with them or we can help with them. Our touch through our hands communicates how we feel inside and our affections to the outside world. You show your intention, how you feel about that person, with touch. When you watch someone touch another person you can see if they value that person through their manner of touching.

> *Mom has slipped down another notch—less responsive, fewer smiles. She stopped trying to walk and is fearful when you push her wheelchair. She is eating less. Well, today was a bright sunny day so I pushed her out onto the patio to cheer her, or me. We sat, me talking, joking, but she just didn't respond. I then thought I saw her tearing up and her nose was running a bit. As she wiped her nose, looking straight ahead, with her eyes glistening, I couldn't keep from crying. At that point something phenomenal happened. With just a glance toward me, we made eye contact, and she reached over and patted my knee with her ice-cold hand. It suddenly felt like I was eight instead of fifty-eight and was being comforted by my loving mother. The bittersweet moment was there and then it was gone.* —A DAUGHTER DEEPLY TOUCHED

Our hands portray our inside state:

* Our love for others
* Our sacrifice for others
* Our suffering for others
* Our anger for another
* Our beliefs about their value as a human being
* Our fears
* Our ignorance

We seek it as children—the touch that shows us affection and security—and I believe we seek it and welcome it as we move to the end of life. We want to sense that the world around us values us. Even in the business of our work and life, we need to be mindful to stop and bring calmness to our body so that our touch communicates time and attention to the person. Touch can and should communicate the following to the Alzheimer's person: You are honored. You are important. You are not alone. You are valued. And we know that you are still there even when you don't look like it or respond like it.

A friend of mine visited her childhood pastor, who had progressive Parkinson's disease. My friend shared how, as a child, she would draw the same picture over and over again for him and he would always hang one of the pictures in his office. They had a special bond. Now her childhood pastor is in a nursing home crumpled in a wheelchair, unable to even open his eyes. On her last visit, she just so happened to bring one of the pictures she had drawn for him. While describing every detail, she placed her hand between his hands. He didn't verbally respond or open his eyes, but a tear came down his cheek. His wife commented on how people didn't visit him anymore because he doesn't respond. This moment was a complete affirmation that he is still in there.

Honor me with touch. Comfort me with touch. Value me with touch. Love me with touch —Teresa Stecker

---

Newfound Touch

Final Moments

Written by Teresa Stecker, R.N., Hospice Nurse, Pastor. (P.S. She's my sister.)

As with all of us, there comes a time when the journey of life comes to an end for the person with Alzheimer's. These final days may go quickly or move slowly. They may be with or without signs of discomfort. As caregivers, we can bring comfort by advocating for the person to be as free of pain and as comfortable as possible. This can be assisted by talking to your physician and/or care community to refer end of life care to the local hospice organization. They specialize in providing comfort to the dying and support to the caregivers.

As an individual moves within hours of death, signs that may be present include restlessness, slower and more irregular breathing, congestion, cold hands and feet, and eyes open. After a few gasping breaths, the journey of life on this earth is complete.

It is beneficial to your family and yourself to formally communicate your wishes regarding your medical treatment at the end of life. It is best for this to be done while you are in good health mentally and physically. These plans should be expressed verbally to your family but also should be written in a living will and a durable power of attorney document. Check with your physician or lawyer regarding these documents.

As I looked at this title, I wondered how I could convey the final moments of joy I have witnessed as a hospice nurse. For most of us, death is viewed as defeat or the end. It is hidden and not talked about but is something we all will face. Let me tell you what I have seen in the final moments of joy while walking through the end-of-life journey with many individuals with Alzheimer's and their families.

I've seen the positive effect of an individual's approaching death; it make others stop and consider their lives. I've seen reconciliation in families. I've seen forgiveness offered where it was denied for several years. I've seen families huddle together in unity, overcoming years of bitter isolation. I've seen laughter ring out over a family joke in the midst of tears. I've seen quiet smiles of remembrance of a mother's last embrace in the midst of sadness. I've seen loyalty and perseverance, where so many times they just wanted to run away.

Sometimes it has been the struggle of feeling like we could have done more or the sense of failure in that relationship. But in thoughtful recollection, we realize we did our best and are only human.

For as we have sought to bring moments of joy to others, it returns. Our own moments of joy come as we rest, remember, and sense the feeling that we did all we knew how to show love. It is our greatest gift and it is the gift that no one can take from us. May you be gentle and loving with yourself as you reflect on the moments of joy you brought to lives that will only repay you in memories and in your inner sense of peace. May that be your moment of joy!

I dressed up as an angel one year for Halloween and walked into this person's room. The lady said, "Are you here to take me home?" I didn't know what to do so I left the room and told the administrator. The administrator encouraged me to go back in the room and sit with her. So I did and I simply said, "I am here. It is okay. I am here." The lady died within five minutes. —A CAREGIVER

When the person says, "I want to go home," they might be asking for permission to leave this world. They will hang on for you if you say, "I will miss you." "I will see you tomorrow." Give them permission to go.

For the past month my mom has been saying that she sees her mom and wants her mom to come inside. I thought I was doing the right thing by replying, "Your mom will be in in a little bit." Last Thursday, I finally understood and said to my mom, "Go get your mom." My mom died within two hours.

When the person is seeing other people who have already passed on, that may be another way of saying it is time to "go home".

I told him, "It's okay to let go. Your work on Earth is done." —A SON

You matter to the last moment of your life, and we will do all we that we can, not only to help you die peacefully, but to live until you die. —DAME CICELY SAUNDERS, FOUNDER OF THE HOSPICE MOVEMENT, LONDON, 1968

Be Gentle

You have learned a lot by simply reading this book. You're going to want to tell your brother because, "He should..." You want to tell your mom because, "She should..." You want to tell other caregivers because, "They should..." Don't go back and "should" on people.

Recognize that each person is doing the best they can with the information they have. The only person you can change after today is...yourself. It's a waste of energy to try to change anyone else. Use that energy to get your hair done or play a round of golf. Yes...GO! When you're feeling better, it simply is better.

You have zero credibility with your family. They might not ask for your advice, BUT...if someone who is an expert on Alzheimer's says it, a family member sees it on the Internet, or a friend hands them this book, it's, "You know what I heard?..." You have been trying for the past two years to get them to "get it." If someone who is a complete stranger says it, then it becomes gospel. Insane phenomenon.

If you are the caregiver...then I know you give and you give and you give. At the end of the day, what do you have to give to yourself? Nothing! Do you think you will get permission from your kids, partner, or person you care for to take care of yourself? Nope. Do you think your brother is going to notice your crabbiness and give you permission to go hang with your friends? Nope. Who is the only one who will give you permission to fit joy into your day? You are! Please give To you...From you.

No one is going to come up to you, a professional caregiver, and say, "You have been working too long. You'd better head home." They will come up to you and ask, "Can you do another shift?" Who is the only one who can say, "No, I am heading home because I am important. My partner is important. My kids are important." Who is the only one who decides what is important? You. And you ARE important!

When my oldest daughter was twelve, I took her out for breakfast on a day I was not traveling and speaking about Alzheimer's. She ordered French toast, at which I commented, "Sid, I didn't even know you liked French toast." She replied in her young wisdom, "Mom if work is all you do, work is all you know." Ouch. The oyster opened, and I got to choose to pick up the pearl. I am a workaholic and giver. I have to make a conscious effort to practice WHO is important. Pause, please. Who is important? —JOLENE

If you put caregiving first in your life, what might you possibly lose in the process? Yourself and the people you love. Is that what anyone wants? No.

Being there when someone needs you is the definition of relationship, and relationships are far from perfect. But accepting each person as they are will make it better. This relationship is no longer healthy when you are losing yourself. Consider your relationship with yourself. Let go of the shoulda, coulda, woulda…you too are doing the best you know how in each moment.

Be Gentle with everyone, and most importantly, Be Gentle with Yourself.

You, yourself, as much as anybody in the entire universe, deserve your love and affection. —THE BUDDHA

Newfound Self-Love

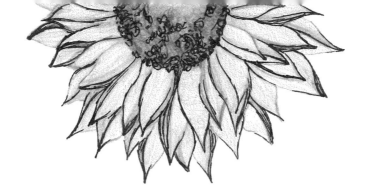

Breathe

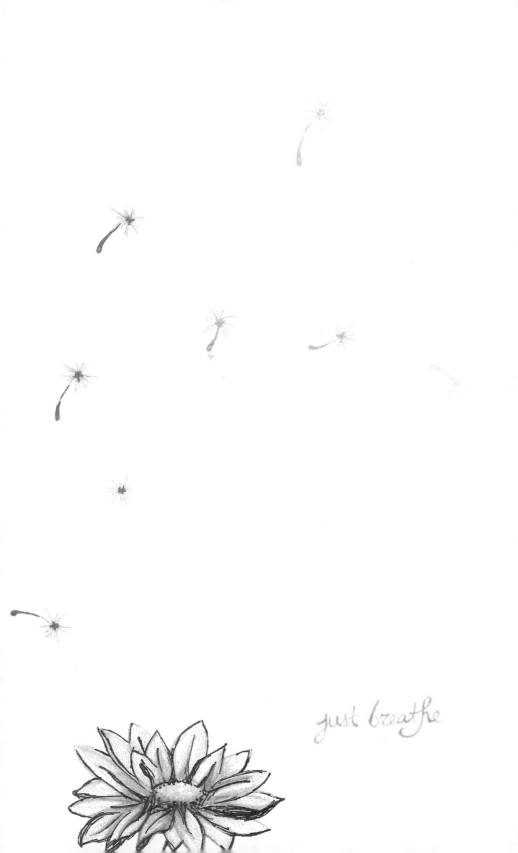

just breathe

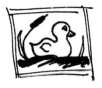

Have you ever sat and watched ducks on a pond? It's almost magical how they move about, seemingly with no effort at all. They appear to be so calm and carefree. The leaves are falling, the breeze is blowing, the sun is shining, and it's a beautiful day. But what are those ducks doing below the surface of the water that we onlookers can't see? Paddling! Paddling! Paddling! (Okay, and pooping.)

Be more like ducks. On the surface, appear calm and carefree, like it's a beautiful day; but when the person asks you, "Where's my mother?," you're paddling, paddling, paddling underneath the surface, where they can't see: "She'll be right back." If you hesitate, or if your tone of voice is uneasy, they won't believe a single word that comes out your mouth. But, if you calmly answer like it's no big deal, then it becomes no big deal. How can you help them to feel like the world is okay in this moment?

Be like a duck…keep calm and unruffled on the surface
but paddle like the devil underneath! —JOLENE

If you forget everything,
try to hang onto these words…

Be like the Duck…

Be like the Sun…

Duck & Sun…

Duck…

Sun…

Duck…

Sun…

One day the Sun in all her radiance was shining high in the sky, when a massive Storm Cloud formed right in front of her. The Storm Cloud said, "I'm more powerful than you! I can raise mighty winds, and pummel the earth with my rain!" The Sun just smiled, which infuriated the Storm Cloud even more. The Storm Cloud said, "See that little boy? Whoever can get his jacket off is the most powerful."

In his pride, the Storm Cloud summoned all of his strength and rolled himself out across the entire skyline, spitting and raining on the little boy, trying to blow off his jacket. The boy held on tighter. At the height of his triumphal display, the Storm Cloud realized he had spent all of his power and he was evaporating away!

The Sun kept shining patiently, radiating her light and warmth. The little boy started to sweat. It was getting hot. The little boy took off his jacket.

The moral of the story is…when you try to force anyone in your life to do what you want them to do, they are going to hold on tighter. But if you are like the Sun—patient, radiant in warmth and light—they are more likely to open up (cooperate). But the real deal breaker is finding the reason they understand. It doesn't matter what you understand…that's going to take therapy for some of you Clouds.

Storm Cloud says: "You haven't bathed in six days!"
Sun says: "Harold is coming tonight. He is handsome!"
Storm Cloud says: "You already had five cups of coffee!"
Sun says: "The coffee is still brewing. Let's see what Bob is doing."
Storm Cloud says: "You live here now. This is your home."
Sun says: "Would you like ice cream before you go?"

When you are like the Sun, you will be more likely to shine through any Storm Cloud that comes your way. —Dustin

or Sunny Duck!

273

Spiritual Strength

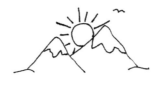

As adolescents, when confronted with an obstacle in our path, we applied our physical strength to it. If we could not push it aside, we would either climb over it or go around it. In our midlife years, we applied our mental strength to it. We would either outthink it or outsmart it. But as we aged into our latter years we realized there were some obstacles in life, some problems, we couldn't push aside, climb over, go around, outthink or outsmart—they could only be endured, which takes spiritual strength.

Alzheimer's disease will defy your physical and mental strength. Only your spiritual strength will empower you enough to make it through to the end. Spend time in prayer, in song, reading, meditating, in service, receiving spiritual guidance, simply connecting with nature, playing an instrument, or doing whatever centers you. Or perhaps just looking at old photos to remind you why you're doing what you're doing.

To make it, you will need great spiritual strength, strong relations with others, and a bagful of tools. I've given you the tools in this book—the rest is up to you.

Yesterday was a bad day here. That is when I raised up my hands and said, "Lord, I turn it over to you again. I can't do it!" Ron is getting to where he thinks I don't know anything. He wants to argue! I won't do it as it makes him so mad! He said he was going to hit me over the head someday! Then five minutes later all was well. I just have to remember to "breathe," take deep breaths!　　　　　　　　　　　　　　　　　　　　—MARVEA

I can do all things through Christ, who strengthens me (Phillipians 4:13). —MY MOM'S VERSE FOR SPIRITUAL STRENGTH

274

The Beginning...

I f I had a penny for every person who said, "I wish I knew this ten years ago," I would be rich. The fact is, you didn't know this ten years ago. Therefore, to feel guilty is unnecessary. If you went back to the moment at which you started to feel guilty and did a replay, given the exact same information, you would do what you did then all over again. Forgive yourself, because in every moment you are doing the best you can.

You have gained a lot of information from this book. Don't try to do it all. Just take one chapter and practice. You can make mistakes all day long and know that tomorrow you get to start fresh because the person doesn't remember the mistakes you made yesterday. Where else do you get so many do-overs?

Forgive yourself in every moment. Begin anew, begin anew...in every moment begin anew.

We ALL need love and care.

How you feel loved is different than how I feel loved, so therefore you are going to want to fill out your own book.

Finish this sentence:
I feel loved when...

Communicate clearly...so the people who love you can start practicing now.

One day I was passing a lady's room and she was calling out, "Jesus, Jesus, Jesus!" I went into her room and said, "I'm not Jesus, but what can I do for you?" She replied, "If you're not Jesus, who is?" —Peace

---

Consider

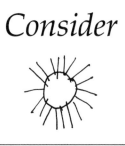

C onsider…people with Alzheimer's can teach us how to live. If they don't remember what happened five minutes ago and they don't know what is going to happen in five minutes…where are they living? In the "now." They need us to meet them there; they demand it. We have an opportunity to be present in each moment, to neither dwell in the past nor worry about the future. Wanting something other than what is right now is the sheer definition of suffering.

People with Alzheimer's, cannot hide, stuff, twist, or change their emotions like we cognitive people can. When they are mad, they are mad. When they are sad, they are sad. When they are scared, they are scared. We get an opportunity to respond to authentic emotions. This practice has the potential to improve all of your relationships. What works with this person will work with your child, friend, partner, or family.

And yes, it is a long goodbye as it allows us to navigate the grieving processing. There becomes an urgency to say all that you want to say as this is a progressive disease; this is a time to heal what is broken. The person will tell you things they never would have told you in their cognitive state.

A lady was sharing how during their entire marriage her husband would be compliant, but now he retorts, "Oh, you think you're smart. You're always so smart." He is now fully expressing himself with her.

They are here to teach us to lighten up. You have no control, especially over another human being. The person will take you on this journey whether you want to go or not. You have a choice: walk with them and embrace their spirit, or resist by staying in the confines of your fears.

Those with Alzheimer's are often a mirror for us to see ourselves in—what we project they reflect. They react to what we are feeling whether we recognize it or not. It is a reminder of how truly interconnected we are.

As I visited Sister Mary Rita in the hospital—a girl after my own heart, a free spirit, a lover of life whom I have watched relish all the little surprises life brings—she looked so tiny, so fragile. I just looked at her and said, "I am you, aren't I?" She nodded and closed her eyes.

When my father was diagnosed with Alzheimer's I could not help but worry that I was looking at my own future. "Will I get Alzheimer's?"

Instead of worrying or being afraid of what will happen, reframe it. We can't do anything with the future, but we can allow care and compassion right now. Live each moment.

We don't get to know. We get to sit in the Unknown, moment by moment. We get to practice being okay with ourselves and the person, as we surrender to the Unknown. We get to feel all of it...joy, kindness, compassion, and anger, guilt, fear, mortality.

Are you curious enough to explore without judgment?
Are you strong enough to let go of all that
"was" and embrace what "is?"
Are you willing to accept all "beings" in
whatever capacity they show up?
Are you ready to accept all, in the face of the unknown?

To believe in...loving a life, loving all, loving fully, loving without limits, without expectation, to love in all ways, and always, in all that we are. —TROY

Newfound Being

Create a Moment ...

E at chocolate ~ recite a poem ~ laugh along ~ bite into fresh strawber-ries ~ whistle a tune ~ talk about goin' fishin' ~ ice cream, ice cream, ice cream ~ go for a walk ~ open a jar of pickles ~ seek shade ~ turn off the TV ~ dance ~ watch the birds ~ picnic in a park ~ bring fried chicken ~ reread the classics ~ play the piano ~ sing out loud ~ hold hands ~ smile a lot ~ catch a firefly ~ drink lemonade ~ listen ~ eat cheeseburgers ~ help them write a letter ~ send mail ~ share a funny story ~ rub lotion into their hands ~ look them in the eye ~ stroke their hair ~ hug them until they let go ~ sing them to sleep ~ notice the clouds ~ pick flowers ~ watch a sunset ~ let them watch you fly a kite ~ hold a baby or hold a doll ~ watch a puppy play ~ visit outside in the breeze ~ snap beans ~ mash potatoes ~ shuck corn ~ peel eggs ~ sit in the sun ~ sneak something from your pocket ~ Bazooka bubblegum ~ lollipops ~ ice pops ~ say "Yes" A LOT ~ look at old photos ~ share a secret ~ eat a Sunday dinner three times a week ~ bite into a gooey cinnamon roll ~ be their friend ~ spritz perfume ~ tell them how terrific they are ~ do what they like to do ~ watch the snow fall ~ nibble on homemade bread with butter ~ nap on a comfy couch ~ let them wear that outfit day after day ~ compliment them (on that outfit) ~ let them take along that worn ugly orange chair ~ tell a joke ~ learn what they have to teach ~ ask for their opinion ~ use your ears more than your mouth ~ let them be right ~ let them take care of you ~ ask them to help ~ thank them for helping the best way they know how ~ be flexible ~ include them ~ accept them as they are ~ be their advocate ~ stay when they are afraid ~ reassure "I'm not going anywhere" ~ be relaxed ~ make them comfortable ~ cover their lap with an afghan ~ touch ~ feel ~ sing "Jesus Loves Me" over and over ~ breathe deeply ~ talk to them even if they don't talk back ~ kiss them on the forehead ~ wave and smile when you part ~ just love them

…Isn't that what you would want?

I want to thank you, Lord,
for being so close to me so far this day.
With your help I haven't been impatient, lost my temper,
or been grumpy, judgmental, or envious of anyone. BUT…
I will be getting out of bed in a minute, and I
think I will really need your help then!
Amen.

I, Jolene Brackey, international speaker on Alzheimer's disease and author of the book *Creating Moments of Joy*, am NOT your teacher. Your experience, in the present moment, is your ONLY teacher.

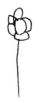

If you are interested in having Jolene Brackey speak to your organization or would like additional training material, please contact:

Enhanced Moments
jolene@enhancedmoments.com
www.enhancedmoments.com

About the Author

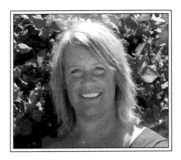

I am blessed beyond measure, grate-full beyond words, and simply humbled by this journey called Life. Affirmation has been found in many ways including this story:

> Two years after I started my business, my mom found a heart I made in Sunday school when I was seven. On that heart I had written: "Love is…knowing Jesus, helping Mom and Dad, helping make the bed, and helping old people."

May we all have sweeter days as we discover our gifts and use them to make a difference in the lives of others.

Joys to you,

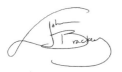